THE FOUNDATIONS OF YOUR PRIVATE PRACTICE
Volume Two: The Complete Book of
Clinical Forms for an Effective Private Practice

Through the years
from Michael
to
Grandpa

THE FOUNDATIONS OF YOUR PRIVATE PRACTICE

Volume Two

The Complete Book of Clinical Forms for an Effective Private Practice

MICHAEL I. GOLD, PH.D.

with

Phyllis Galbraith, M.A.
Jean Yingling, M.A., MFCC

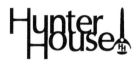

For further information contact:
Hunter House Inc., Publishers
P.O. Box 2914
Alameda, CA 94501-0914

All the names and incidents used for the case history in this book are fictitious.

The authors are grateful for permission received to reprint from the following: "Client's Bill of Rights" from *The California Therapist*, the publication of the California Association of Marriage and Family Therapists, Nov/Dec 1989, used with permission; "Guidelines for Patients Entering Group Therapy" adapted from Ann Spadone Jacobson, Ph.D., Psychologist; "Ethical Principles," American Association for Marriage and Family Therapy, AAMFT Code of Ethics. Washington DC, American Association of Marriage and Family Therapy, 1991, pp. 1–12. Copyright © 1991 by American Association of Marriage and Family Therapy, reprinted with permission; the Suspected Child Abuse Report form on page 84, from the California Department of Justice, Missing and Exploited Children Program, reprinted with permission.

Library of Congress Cataloging-in-Publication Data
The foundations of your private practice.
p. cm.
Includes bibliographic references and index.
Contents: v. 1. The building of your private practice / by Michael I. Gold with Colette McDougall — v. 2. The complete book of clinical forms for an effective private practice / by Michael I. Gold with Phyllis A. Galbraith, Jean Yingling.
ISBN 0-89793-124-6 (v. 1 : hardcover): $29.95 — ISBN 0-89793-125-4 (v. 2 : hardcover): $74.95 — ISBN (invalid) 0-89793-126-2 (forms): $50.00
1. Psychiatry—Practice. 2. Psychiatry—Practice—Forms. I. Gold, Michael I.
[DNLM: 1. Practice Management, Medical. 2. Psychotherapy. W 80 F771 1993]
RC465.5.F68   1993
6616.89'0068—dc20
DNLM/DLC
for Library of Congress   93–12015

Manufactured in the United States of America

9 8 7 6 5 4 3 2 1   First edition

Project Credits

Project managers: Lisa E. Lee (editorial)   Paul J. Frindt (production)
Cover designs by Tamra Goris Graphics and Jil Weil Designs
Book design by *Qalagraphia*
Copyeditors: Mali Apple, Janja Lalich
Proofreader: Susan Burckhard
Production Assistance: María Jesús Aguiló Pérez
Marketing: Corrine M. Sahli
Customer Support: Sharon R. A. Olson, James Rachogan
Fulfillment: A & A Quality Shipping Services
Publisher: Kiran S. Rana
Set in Palatino and Goudy Sans by 847 Communications, Alameda, CA
Printed by Publishers Press, Salt Lake City

Ordering

Individuals may order additional copies of the two volumes or the forms packages using the order form at the end of the book. Hunter House books are available at special discounts for sales promotions, organizations, premiums, fundraising, and for educational use. For details please contact:

Special Sales Department
Hunter House Inc., Publishers
P.O. Box 2914
Alameda, CA 94501-0914
Phone: (510) 865-5282   Fax: (510) 865-4295

Trade bookstores in the U.S. and Canada please contact:

Publishers Group West
4065 Hollis Street, Box 8843
Emeryville CA 94608
Phone: (800) 788-3123 Fax: (510) 658-1834

Table of Contents

List of Forms

All the forms preceded by an X are included
as reproducible photocopy masters in the forms
pack that accompanies this volume.

X   Authorization to Obtain Confidential Information   74

X   Consent for Release of Confidential Information   76

X   Clinical Consultations   78

X   Life-Threatening Behavior Scale   80

     Suspected Child Abuse Report   85

X   Certificate to Return to Work or School   87

X   Fees for Depositions and Court Appearances   89

X   Assignment of Lien   91

Chapter 5: Filling in the Client's Background

X   Confidential Personal History I   94

X   Confidential Personal History II   99

X   Confidential Vocational History   108

X   Confidential Chemical (Substance Use) History   113

X   Confidential Sexual History   127

Chapter 6: Writing Your Reports

     Mental Health Treatment Report   135

     Psychological Report   143

     Psychiatric Evaluation   155

Important Notice

The material in this book is intended to provide a review of information regarding setting up a private psychotherapy practice. Every effort has been made to provide accurate and dependable information. The contents of this book have been carefully reviewed by experts in the field. However, professional therapists have differing opinions and ways of approaching the practice of therapy, therefore the information presented herein should be regarded as the expertise of the authors.

The publisher, authors, editors, and reviewers cannot be held responsible for any error, omission, or dated material. The author and publisher assume no responsibility for any outcome of the use of any of these procedures in setting up a private practice.

If you have a question concerning your own practice, or about the legal appropriateness or application of the procedures described in this book, consult your attorney.

Although many state and national agencies and associations have been extremely helpful in providing information and resource material for this book, the reader should be informed that the appearance of materials and/or the inclusion of information does not represent any agency or association approval of the contents of this book.

Acknowledgments

I would like to thank the many people that helped make this two-volume publication a reality. Thank you to Ted Pedersen; Emil Soorani, M.D.; Vera David, Ph.D.; Wyler Greene, Ph.D.; Harold Foster, M.A.; Harvey Mindess, Ph.D.; Mary Proteau; Richard Marsh, Ph.D.; Bob Martinez; Mali Apple, Janja Lalich and Kate McKinley; the State of California Department of Consumer Affairs and its agencies; the American Psychiatric Association; the Associations of Marriage and Family Therapists; the dozens of civil servants in local, county, and state agencies; and to the tireless people at Hunter House, from publisher Kiran Rana, production manager, Paul Frindt, and editor Lisa Lee, to assistant to the publisher Corrine Sahli; and finally, to my friend and colleague, John Ranyard.

Thank you.

Michael I. Gold
Hermosa Beach, CA
January 1994

Introduction

"Render Unto Caesar..."

I have been a practicing psychotherapist since 1968, and the information and forms in this book are the result of what I have learned in those years of experience. Like many others, I learned through the painful process of trial and error. By giving you the benefit of my labors, I hope to make your life a little easier.

From my first day of clinical practice, I felt I knew how to render unto God. But, as I quickly realized, I also needed to learn how to render unto Caesar.

"Rendering unto God" should not be taken as a religious statement. However, I continue to be amazed at the "magic" that must take place between a client and a therapist for healing, clarity, and affirmation to occur. "Rendering unto Caesar" implies that I have a fiduciary responsibility to and for my client in dealing with state boards, insurance companies, subpoenas, testimony, reports—all those aspects of life that require "proof" of my craft.

The art of being a psychotherapist is the art of loving another human being. If "work is love made visible," as Kahlil Gibran suggests, then as practitioners of the healing arts, we have equal responsibilities to render unto God *and* to Caesar. The technical, and at times bureaucratic, aspects of our work are part and parcel of what we do and the reason for my sharing with you some ways of making your love for your clients visible.

Some of the forms in this book attend to the busywork of being a practitioner. Others, such as the Mental Status Examination, are a necessary aid to quantifying both training and intuitive clinical skills.

With the help of colleagues and other professionals in various disciplines, I have organized these forms with an eye toward simplicity and convenience. It is my hope that some of these forms will stimulate an area of clinical consideration that has gone unfocused in your day-to-day practice. Further, it is my aim that these forms will enhance your confidence in areas and aspects of clinical work that too many clinicians have found to be not only tedious but, at times, frightening.

If they achieve even a small portion of these goals, the thousands of hours that went into the development of these forms will have been worthwhile.

A Personal Discovery

Sometime during the first five years of my private practice I was informed by a client that I would be receiving a questionnaire from his insurance company. He requested that I fill out the form as soon as I received it and return it to the insurance company. I agreed and soon forgot about it. Within two weeks the questionnaire arrived.

The insurance company forms required me to record the dates of our consultations, my diagnosis, and my prognosis relating to the future possible disability of my client. Consulting my records to check the dates of consultation and filling out the form took about 10 minutes. As I was folding the questionnaire to put it in the envelope, I noticed an attachment at the top of the last form. It was a check.

The check was made out to me and presigned by the insurance company's representative. The amount of the check was blank. A statement on the check read, "Not valid for over $25,000."

After larcenous thoughts, I knew this must be a mistake, so I called the physician's assistance number that was provided. When I informed the insurance advisor that her company had mistakenly sent me a blank check, I will never forget her response. "It's not a mistake. You just fill in the correct amount. You're the doctor."

"You're the doctor." I was stunned. I sat staring at this check which could pay every bill I had in the world and leave me enough money to go to Europe for a long time.

"You're the doctor." Then (I remember this as clear as if it were happening as I write this) I said aloud, "*I'm* the doctor."

"You're the doctor" had been magically transformed into *I'm the doctor.*

Forgetting the idiocy of our insurance system, I realized that the assistant on the other end of the line had taught me something that I had not learned in 22 years of education, 3 years of internship, and 5 years of clinical practice: I'm the doctor.

I filled in the amount on the check for $25 and mailed it.

When you receive an insurance form, or your first subpoena, it is important for you to remember, whether you have an M.D., Ph.D., MFCC, M.A., M.S., MSW, MCSW, or whatever after your name, that *you* are the doctor. Go ahead, say it aloud: I'm the doctor.

Most of all, remember this: All the rewards and all the concomitant responsibilities are housed in that statement. Change my forms. Don't use the ones you don't want to use. Fill out, or have your client fill out, the forms you decide are in the best interest of *your* practice, *your* clients, and *your*self. Bad forms, like bad laws, have a tendency to "stay on the books" beyond their usefulness or even their intent. But remember that, above all, with all its joys and all its terrors, you're the doctor.

How to Use This Book

There are two parts to Volume Two. The first section is a walk-through of all the forms. I have used a representative client as a working example so that you can see how the forms are used in daily practice.

Each chapter begins with an overview explaining the purpose of the forms in that section. Then sample forms are presented completed as they might be by either the client or you. In addition, some personal notations are included, which comment on a particular clinical process reflected in a form.

Also included are a number of sample reports that have been prepared from information collected from the forms relating to the sample patient. These reports will guide you in preparing your own professional reports.

In demonstrating how to use these forms, I have drawn from my own practice as well as from the clinical practices of other practitioners. Based on my research, I have created a composite patient/client named Michelle Silver.

Through the travails of our mythical Michelle, while she goes through everything in the book as a patient, I hope to put *you* through everything in the book as a therapist. From the initial Referral Tracking Sheet through the different reporting forms to the reports compiled from these forms, I have attempted to take this poor person—and you—through the clinical jungle.

You will observe Michelle as she develops through the use of all the forms and formats and becomes a real person. I want to demonstrate to you that a client can emerge on paper as well as in session. At the same time, I have tried to keep her diagnostically within the confines of an ordinary person. The examples used inhe text are a composite of the responses gleaned from the clinical and legal experiences of many competent professionals.

Even though all the forms are used with Michelle, in the history of my practice I have never used *all* my forms with a single person. You may find that due to the nature of your practice you will rarely, if ever, use all the forms discussed and provided here.

The second section of this volume is a complete, ready-to-print collection of the forms which you can reproduce and use in your own practice. This "packet," though, is more than just a collection of ready-to-use fill-in-the-blank forms. It embodies a comprehensive process of capturing information—a process that will enable you to provide the best professional service to your clients.

If you are charging more than $35 per session, this packet of forms will save you thousands of dollars. It is designed to be "a private practice in a box." If you only use a form once in your entire clinical practice, it will save you hours of time.

As you will note throughout, the terms *patient* and *client* are used intermittently. (Bless the memory of Dr. Carl Rogers.) Whether to use *client* or *patient* on any given form or within the context of the formatted reports was a constant and ongoing professional discussion among us, the writers of this book. In Volume One, we exclusively used *client*. In this Volume we decided to use *client* and *patient* intermittently to keep the debate alive. The nature of your practice will probably determine which word you prefer. If, for the purposes of your practice, you wish to alter either term please remember once again the caveat of this work: you're the doctor.

A Special Note Concerning DSM IV...

Please note that some of the forms are directly tied to the DSM-III-R, ICD-9, and presently used Current Procedural Terminology (CPT) codes. The changes that are going to occur in the DSM-IV as related to the ICD-10 have been researched. The new diagnostic formats and numbering system will be added once they are available and current, and through arrangement with the publisher it will be possible to receive the updated formats.

1

Before the Client Arrives
Forms to Be Used
Before Counseling Begins

This chapter recognizes the "paper hassle" requirements of opening a private practice. Ordinarily, the state will license you to practice your craft—counseling or psychology—while the city and county will be interested in you as a business venture.

More and more states are requiring forms that are generated by state agencies. Practicalities obviously do not allow for the printing here of all the forms necessary for beginning a private practice in your state and city. But, using California as an example, an assortment of sample forms is included, such as the forms necessary for notifying the state of the employment of interns, the weekly record of interns' experience hours, and city and county forms such as business license applications. You can obtain specific copies of the forms required in your area by contacting the city clerk or state licensing agency.

If you haven't already, you will discover that colleges and universities, state agencies, local government agencies, and even state and national associations will often have contradictory information. Our profession is in an enormous state of flux and, with the inevitable advent of national health insurance, we can expect a plethora of new forms for reimbursement of our services. The message I want to communicate is simply this: at times, you will need to call four people to get one answer.

At Antioch University in Los Angeles, where I teach in the graduate psychology school, the director of placement has developed an expertise in aiding students, beginning clinicians, and supervisors in writing appropriate letters and using how-to tips for filling out forms. With a little searching you can find a similar person at a state agency or local university psychology department who can aid you with these processes. Offering a small fee for that person to meet with you regarding forms can be informative and cost effective.

Business License Applications
For complying with local business laws

On the following pages are samples of license applications for the Los Angeles area. The business license application and the home occupation permit application illustrate the difference in the forms you will be required to complete depending on whether you run your practice from your home or from an office away from home.

These forms may seem lengthy compared to those of other cities. They serve to illustrate how extensive forms can get.

Do not confuse business licenses with state licensure. State licensure refers to the credentialing of a professional for the purpose of practicing his or her art, craft, or profession in a public or private setting. States typically maintain control over the standards necessary to obtain a given license or credential. A business license is generally issued by the city or township in which you intend to practice, and involves money paid to the local government to fund local public services.

Most cities charge a fee through the city clerk's office for professional services rendered in the city. Basic fees range from $15 to $750. In addition to these fees, the city may exact an additional tax based on the gross amount of money the business earns. To compute these earnings I use the dollar amounts from my income tax forms, since the city has a right to verify earnings. The additional earnings tax is usually small (e.g., one tenth of 1%).

The city can also assess your inventory. Your books, office furniture, and even office decor can be assessed, and a property tax based on that assessment must be paid. Whether you are paying for a business license, a home permit, or your inventory, there is generally an upper limit to the amount you have to pay.

If you are considering not applying for a license or permit, remember that there are city employees who can literally walk into waiting rooms of professionals to see whether the permit or license is in public

BUSINESS LICENSE APPLICATION

SAMPLE

The Undersigned Hereby Requests a License to Conduct Business in the City of: __Yourville__

Part I Applicant to Answer all Questions in this Section

1. License Number	2. Application Number

3. Business Name or DBA *GEORGE R. JONES, Ph.D., MFCC*

4. Corporate Name (if different from above) *NONE*

5. Business Address *929 W. MAIN BLVD., STE 101, LOS ANGELES, CA 90000*	6. Business Phone *(213) 555-7927*

7. Mailing Address *SAME*

8. Description of Business *PSYCHOTHERAPY PRACTICE*

Check if Applicable: ☐ Corp/Admin. Headquarters ☑ Professional ☐ Manufacturing ☐ Service ☐ Retail ☐ Wholesale

9. Driver's License No. *C3333333*	10. Social Security No. *999-99-9999*	11. State Sales Tax No. *SAME AS 10*	12. Federal ID No. *SAME AS 10*
13. State Contractor Lic. No. *NONE*	14. State ID No. *H21032*	15. Business Start Date in *3-1-94*	16. SIC No.

17. If Sole Ownership, Enter Name, Address and Phone:
GEORGE R. JONES, 76 OCEAN AVE., LOS ANGELES, CA 90000   *(213) 555-4892*

18. If Corporation or Partnership, Complete the Following: *N/A*   ☐ Partnership   ☐ Corporation

Names of Partners or Principal Officers	Title	Home Address	Home Phone
N/A			
1.			
2.			
3.			

Signature of Person Making Application *George R. Jones*   Date *1-4-94*

Part II

If your business is located in Yourville you must answer the following questions:

1. Are chemicals used (other than consumer products)? ☐ Yes ☑ No

2. Are any of the above chemicals stored in quantities greater than 55 gallons, 500 pounds or 200 cubic feet to compressed gas in aggregate quantities? ☐ Yes ☑ No

3. Are any of the above chemicals discharged into the city sewer or storm drain? ☐ Yes ☑ No

4. Enter the number of persons working (20 hours or more per week) at business: *1*

Part III Optional Question

The following question will help the City operate its Women and Minoritites Business Enterprises Program but is not a requirement for obtaining a Yourville Business License.

1. Is your business owned and controlled by women or minority persons? ☐ Yes ☑ No

(If yes, and you wish to be considered as a potential supplier of goods or services to the City, complete a "WMBE Directory" Enrollment Form and Affidavit and submit it with your Business License Application.)

Part IV For Official Use Only

License Fee	Penalty	Police Permit Fee
Planning App/HO Fee	Fire Permit/Fingerprinting Fee	Assessment/Other Fee

Acceptance of payment does not constitute approval of business license. Authorization to conduct business is not granted until

Form FPP-1-1/1-rev2/94 ©1994 GMS. Do not reproduce. For orders call (510) 865-5282, fax (510) 865-4295.

Home Occupation Permit Application

SAMPLE

City of Yourville
Land Use and Transportation Management Department
Planning and Zoning Division
Telephone (*213*) *555-0204*

PERMIT APPLICATION FEE: $____

| For Office Use Only: |
| HO# _____ LICENSE# _____ |

NAME *GEORGE R. JONES* _____ PHONE *(213) 555-2742*
ADDRESS *15 GREEN BLVD., LOS ANGELES, CA 90002* _____
TYPE OF BUSINESS *PSYCHOTHERAPY PRACTICE* _____
BUSINESS NAME *N/A* _____

THE FOLLOWING QUESTIONS MUST BE ANSWERED IN FULL. Please type or print all responses.

1. People and activities involved: *THERAPISTS AND CLIENTS;*
   COUNSELING AND THERAPY

2. Materials and equipment stored or used: *SIMPLE OFFICE SUPPLIES:*
   DUP. MACHINE, FILE CABINET, FAX

3. Methods and hours of operation: *8 AM – 8 PM*

4. Parking and use of vehicles: *IN DRIVEWAY*

5. Physical alterations to the home: *NONE*

> Please complete both sides of this form as completely as possible. The Zoning Administrator may approve a Home Occupation Permit only when all of the following findings can be made and satisfied in an affirmative manner.

1. Will the home occupation be conducted entirely within a dwelling or accessory building? ☑Yes ☐No

2. Will any horticultural activities be conducted outdoors and within the rear one-half of the parcel? ☐Yes ☑No

3. Will any portion of any required garage or carport be used for home occupation purposes? ☑Yes ☐No

4. Will the home occupation alter the appearance of the dwelling unit such that the structure may be recognized as serving a nonresidential use (either by color, materials or construction, lighting, signs, sounds or noises, vibrations, etc.)? ☐Yes ☑No

5. Will there be sales of goods or displays of goods on the premise? ☐Yes ☑No

6. Will there be signs other than the address and name of any resident? ☐Yes ☑No

7. Will there be outdoor advertising which identifies the home occupation by street address? ☐Yes ☑No

Form FPP-2-1/2-rev2/94 ©1994 GMS. Do not reproduce. For orders call (510) 865-5282, fax (510) 865-4295.

8. Will any commercial vehicles be used for delivery of materials, with the exception of reasonable courier services, to or from the premises?   ☐ Yes ☑ No

9. Will no more than one vehicle larger than a ¾ ton truck be used in connection with a home occupation?   ☐ Yes ☑ No

10. Will on-site parking for any vehicle used in connection with the home occupation be provided in addition to parking required for residents?   ☑ Yes ☐ No

11. Please list activities conducted, and equipment, material or hazardous materials used: ☐ Yes ☑ No

_____

_____

12. Will the fire safety or occupancy classifications of the premises be changed because of the home occupancy?   ☐ Yes ☑ No

13. Will the use create or cause hazards or nuisances due to noise, dust, vibration, odors, smoke, glare, electrical interference, or other reasons?   ☐ Yes ☑ No

14. Will any employees, other than residents of the dwelling unit, be allowed to work, gather, or congregate on the premises in connection with a home occupation with the exception of baby-sitters or domestic staff?   ☐ Yes ☑ No

15. Where the person conducting the home occupation serves as an agent or intermediary between outside suppliers and outside customers, will all articles, except for samples, be received, stored, and sold directly to customers at an off-premises location?   ☐ Yes ☑ No

16. Will there be any storage of material or mechanical equipment not recognized as being part of a normal household or hobby use?   ☐ Yes ☑ No

17. Will there be any excessive or unsightly storage of materials or supplies, indoors or outdoors, for purposes other than those permitted in the residential district in which it is located?   ☐ Yes ☑ No

18. Will the home occupation generate pedestrian or vehicular traffic beyond that ordinarily generated in the residential district in which it is located?   ☐ Yes ☑ No

19. Will the home occupation result in excess use of utilities and public facilities in amounts greater than those normally provided for residential use?   ☐ Yes ☑ No

Please note that the Home Occupation Permit shall be valid only for the person to whom it is issued and shall be void when that person moves from the dwelling unit or discontinues the business.

I HEREBY CERTIFY UNDER PENALTY OF PERJURY THAT THIS INFORMATION IS CORRECT, AND I AGREE to conduct the Home Occupation in conformity with Municipal Code and as stated in response to the above questions. I understand that a separate Business License must be obtained from the City License Division.

Applicant's Signature: _George R. Jones_   Date: _2-4-94_

Driver's License Number: _C3333333_   State: _CA_

Approved: _____   Date: _____
City Planning Staff

Form FPP-2-2/2-rev2/94 ©1994 GMS. Do not reproduce. For orders call (510) 865-5282, fax (510) 865-4295.

view. If you are caught practicing without a permit and license, you will generally have to pay back fees for the number of years you have been practicing, plus a percentage fine for not having a license, and interest on the money owed. Depending on your location, this can be a sizable amount of money.

Remember that you may need to pay a percentage of your total income. Don't be shocked when you receive from the licensing bureau a license renewal form that looks like an income tax form. Generally one page in length, it will be easy to fill out. It will always include a formula for determining how much you must pay for the coming year's license.

Some cities require you to show up in person when initiating a new business. Other cities allow you to handle the process entirely by mail. Call your city clerk's office, which will direct you to the appropriate person who can answer all your questions.

Cities want your business, and they tend to treat applicants for business licenses efficiently and courteously. Although you may never need to write a letter of complaint, should the need arise, write a succinct and direct letter of complaint addressed to the city manager of your municipality. It will produce quick results and perhaps an apology. Remember: you're the doctor.

Now that you have filled out all your business forms, displayed your licenses on the wall, and swept up the hair you pulled out in the process of getting through all of this, it is time to prepare to meet your first client.

Helplines
For reaching potential clients

Before we can meet with our clients, we must have clients to meet. It is unlikely that clients will beat a path to your door—unless they are aware of your availability. And it is your first task to make them aware of your existence.

Helplines, places where people can call to get help, exist in all parts of the country. Lists of helplines are useful both as handouts and as recruiting tools for reaching potential clients. While our information-rich society is overwhelmed with data, it is often difficult to unearth the right source for a particular need. By compiling and distributing this kind of source information, you become a valuable asset. And, because you attach your name to it, you advertise your availability as a therapist in a subtle yet effective way.

National Helplines

Abortion Hotline	(800) 772-9100
AIDS Prevention Center	(800) 322-8911
AIDS Hotline	(800) 551-2728
Al-Anon, Family Groups	(212) 301-7240
Alcoholics Anonymous	(212) 686-1100
Alzheimer's and Related Disorders Association	(800) 621-0379
American Cancer Society	(800) ACS-2345
American Diabetes Association	(800) 232-3472
American Humane Association, Children's Division	(800) 277-5242
Battered Women's Task Force	(414) 466-1660
Birth Control Information Line	(800) 468-3637
Bulimia/Anorexia 24-Hour Crisis Line	(800) 762-3334
Cancer Information Service	(800) 4-CANCER
Child Abuse Hotline	(800) 422-4453
Council on Alcoholism and Drug Dependence, info and referral	(212) 206-6770
Down's Syndrome Society Hotline	(800) 221-4602
Eating Disorder Hotline	(800) 233-5450
Emotions Anonymous	(612) 647-9712
Gamblers Anonymous	(213) 386-8789
The Grief Recovery Institute	(800) 445-4808
National Headache Foundation	(800) 843-2256
National Legal Aid and Defender Association	(202) 452-0620
Narcotics Anonymous	(818) 780-3951
National Mental Health Consumer's Association	(215) 735-2465
Parents Anonymous	(800) 421-0353
Planned Parenthood Federation	(212) 541-7800
Runaway Hotline	(800) 231-6946
VD National Hotline	(800) 277-8922

_____   _____

_____   _____

_____   _____

Local Helplines

Al-Anon, Family Groups   _____

Alcoholics Anonymous   _____

Animal Rescue and Care Center   _____

Apartment Rental Service   _____

Battered Women's Resource   _____

Child Abuse, shelter care   _____

Childcare Resource   _____

Community Library Information   _____

Drug Counseling   _____

Meals on Wheels   _____

Narcotics Anonymous   _____

Planned Parenthood   _____

Senior Information   _____

Teen Clinic   _____

Tenant-Landlord Information   _____

Others:

_____   _____

_____   _____

_____   _____

_____   _____

_____   _____

_____   _____

Provided by:

YOUR NAME AND
PHONE NUMBER
HERE

Some people give away calendars. I have found it effective to collect and give away the phone numbers of helplines. For example, Los Angeles County publishes a Department of Social Services Directory that I purchase each year. I glean other phone numbers from suicide prevention centers, local and city newspapers, and professional magazines. I gather this information and disseminate it freely—always being careful to add my name and telephone number to the handout. I not only become a helpline myself, but I am also contacted for professional services by persons who receive my handouts.

Your private practice will be enhanced, professionally and economically, by your being available as an information resource for clients, their families, and their friends. Have on reserve a referral library consisting of clinicians, agencies, and helplines. When you refer someone to a helpline or another professional, you are building a reputation that is not narcissistically focused. This free auxiliary service can pay off handsomely in the recruitment of future clients.

The sample helpline list includes a page of national helplines and a page for local numbers. I believe that disseminating such a list not only spreads good will, but is one of our professional responsibilities.

Handouts
For advertising and promoting your services

The following passage is something I received at an Alcoholics Anonymous meeting. When I inquired about its authorship, I was told, "It's just one of those things that has floated around the meetings for years."

Letting Go

To let go doesn't mean to stop caring.
>   It means I can't do it for someone else.
To let go is not to cut myself off.
>   It is the realization that I cannot control another.
To let go is not to enable.
>   It is allowing learning from natural consequences.
To let go is to admit powerlessness.
>   The outcome is not in my hands.
To let go is not to try to change or blame another.
>   I can only change myself.

To let go is not to care for another.
        It is to care about another.
To let go is not to judge.
        It is allowing another to be a human being.
To let go is not to be in the middle, arranging all the outcomes.
        It is allowing others to effect their own outcome.
To let go is not to be protective.
        It is to permit another to face reality.
To let go is not to deny.
        It is to accept.
To let go is not to nag, scold or argue.
        It is to search out my own shortcomings and correct them.
To let go is not to adjust everything to my desires.
        It is to take each day as it comes and to cherish the moment.
To let go is not to criticize and regulate anyone.
        It is to try to become what I dream I can be.
To let go is not to regret the past.
        It is to grow and live for the future.
To let go is to fear less and love more.
Face it! Embrace it! Erase it!

Look for this kind of material within the context of your practice. It exists. Print handouts on your personalized stationery, or add your name to them to them in some other way. Your handouts will be useful in your practice and for giving away during lectures or speeches.

Whenever you speak, especially in areas adjacent to your practice, leave the audience with something they can take with them that includes your name and phone number. Acknowledge the source or resource, and pass it on to the audience as something that fits within the context of your speech.

Handouts of this type serve many purposes, two of which come to mind immediately: you don't have to reinvent the wheel, and they are a form of sharing and advertising.

Membership Applications
For applying to professional organizations

Following is a short list of the national organizations that represent the majority of mental health professionals, excluding clergy. These organizations, after checking your qualifications, will be eager for your membership. When some form of national health insurance is implemented, these organizations will perform the duties of political action committees (PACs) and will act as our representatives in helping our profession to be included or excluded from national health insurance.

American Psychological Association
750 First Street NE
Washington DC 20002-4242
(202) 336-5500

American Psychiatric Association
1400 K Street NW
Washington DC 20005
(202) 682-6068

American Association of Marriage and Family Therapy
1100 17th Street NW, 10th Floor
Washington DC 20036
(202) 452-0109

National Association of Social Workers
7981 Eastern Avenue
Silver Spring MD 20910
(202) 408-8600

Aside from developing ethical standards, these organizations provide forums for professional debate and can provide you with sizable discounts in insurance plans, from disability to professional liability.

Many of these organizations raise funds or request money from members who wish to support specific political agendas. Such activities give you the opportunity to accept or reject association policies depending on your beliefs and opinions.

If you do not wish to join national organizations, at least consider joining your state and local organizations. Information ranging from new laws affecting your profession, to PACs acting at the state and local levels, to the mundane but absolutely necessary advertising of goods and services including office rental, is provided through their publications and mailings. To neglect the political necessity of being represented as a profession is an abdication of your potential to effect change that may benefit your clients and you in the near and distant future. Join. Join. Join!

Some state and local associations are affiliated with national organizations. By joining one of these organizations, such as the local American

Psychological Association, you are automatically affiliated with the larger organization. In some cases you must first be a member of the national or state organization to get a discounted membership with the local affiliate.

Look in the yellow pages for local organizations first. State associations tend to be listed in the large city directories. Then call or write the state and national associations. Ask for a copy of their newsletter or magazine to see if the information from that organization is what you want.

Sometimes by joining one association you can receive benefits from another. For example, if you are a member of the California Association of Marriage and Family Therapists (CAMFT), you can get professional liability insurance through the American Association of Marriage and Family Therapy at a discounted rate—in this case, a 50% discount. It costs $100 a year to be a member of CAMFT. This alone can save you $150.

Referral Tracking Sheet
For initial telephone consultations

In today's market, private practice clinicians need to reinforce their suppliers and providers. They should also be aware of which providers give the greatest number of referrals and what kind of referrals they send. Keep a referral tracking sheet next to the phone where you receive incoming messages.

Keep a referrer's file next to your phone as well. When making initial phone contact with a prospective client, pull the file sheet, alphabetized by last name. Ask the prospective client, "Who referred you?" and add the referral source to your file if it is not listed.

At the completion of the phone call, pull the referral tracking sheet and add the client's name. Then send a referral acknowledgment letter to the source of the referral. Copy the letter format supplied here in your own handwriting, or have it redesigned in the form of a thank-you greeting card to suit your taste.

Note that the comment section of the referral tracking sheet is about the referral source, not the referred client.

Date: *12-15-92*	**REFERRAL TRACKING SHEET**	Page No. *1*

Referral Source:	*YOUNG* *ROBERT* *M.D.*	Page No. *1*
	Last Name First Name	

Address: *2201 CENTER BLVD.*
LOS ANGELES, CA 90000

Relationship to Clinician:
☐ Client
☑ Medical
☐ Legal
☐ Friend
☐ Other

Telephone: *(213) 444-3333*

Comments:

TENDS TO REFER COURT CASES (PTSD — DEPRESSION — GENERALLY PATIENTS ARE MEDICATED BY HIM). PAY SPECIAL ATTENTION TO CLINICAL NOTATIONS DURING THERAPY.

Name of Referred Client: *KARA SHAH*	Date: *8-25-92*
Address: *222 SHERMAN BLVD., SANTA MONICA, CA 90404*	
Telephone: *(213) 555-2121*	
Referral acknowledgment sent: ☑	Date: *8-25-92*
Name of Referred Client: *CRYSTAL LANSING*	Date: *11-13-92*
Address: *7999 RUDDER PLACE, SHERMAN OAKS, CA 91376*	
Telephone: *(818) 555-1212*	
Referral acknowledgment sent: ☑	Date: *11-13-92*
Name of Referred Client: *FRED TUCKER*	Date: *1-27-93*
Address: *26 NAVAL DRIVE, STUDIO CITY, CA 91210*	
Telephone: *(818) 555-3434*	
Referral acknowledgment sent: ☑	Date: *1-27-93*
Name of Referred Client:	Date:
Address:	
Telephone:	
Referral acknowledgment sent: ☐	Date:
Name of Referred Client:	Date:
Address:	
Telephone:	
Referral acknowledgment sent: ☐	Date:

Referral Acknowledgment Letter
For acknowledgment of professional resources

When I receive an agency or professional referral, I find it useful as well as courteous to acknowledge the person who initiated the referral with a brief and simple thank-you note. The referral acknowledgment letter, Format A, is a quick and convenient way of doing this.

I have also developed my own informal stationery (see referral acknowledgment letter, Format B). This standard 8½x11 sheet of paper is another way to send personal thank-you notes and acknowledgments of service referred by agencies or individuals. If you fold the Format B letter in half horizontally (so that the printing remains on the outside), then turn the form so that "from the mind of" is in the upper left-hand corner, then make another horizontal fold in half, you will see a card designed for these occasions.

The recipient, upon opening the envelope, finds one of my favorite quotes from Albert Einstein. Unfolding the card, the recipient then reads my personal message.

Design something that reflects your personality and your style. Pick the color and texture of the envelope and the card. Try to design your card to require printing on only one side of the paper, which will save on printing costs. Otherwise, use this idea as a springboard for your own imagination.

Dear _____,

I just want to take a moment to thank you for referring _____. I appreciate the trust and confidence you have in my services.

Each referral is a quiet affirmation of my work. I thank you for giving that to me!

Best wishes,

Referral Acknowledgment Letter, Format A

MAN IS HERE for the sake of other men—above all, for those upon whose smile and well-being our own happiness depends, and also for the countless unknown souls with whose fate we are connected by a bond of sympathy. Many times a day I realize how much my own outer and inner life is built upon the labors of my fellow-men, both living and dead, and how earnestly I must exert myself in order to give in return as much as I have received.

—ALBERT EINSTEIN

from the mind of Michael Gelb

Referral Acknowledgment Letter, Format B

Employment Notification for MFCC Intern, Weekly Summary of Hours, and Sample Letter of Agreement
For complying with state statutes

I first applied for my psychologist's license in 1970. My application was rejected on the grounds that my clinical training began on September 13, 1967, and in order to be granted a license, my training would have had to begin on September 11—only two days earlier. I was further informed that I would have to return to school, take many courses over, and repeat 4,000 hours of clinical training. Some day I will write a book entitled *Crime and Punishment, or Attaining Licensure.*

I trusted my supervisor, my university, and the letter I had received from the state licensing board. I did not know at the time that I was interning on a grandfather (time limited) clause; I didn't even know what a grandfather clause was. Either my supervisors or my university didn't know or didn't provide me with that information.

You can suffer needlessly if you do not contact your state licensing agency or professional association about licensing requirements. At the time I applied, both organizations had brochures and newsletters that explained the change of licensing requirements that were essential in obtaining my license.

A contractual relationship must exist between the supervisor and the agency where the internship is being performed, and between the intern and the agency. This ensures that the agency has recognized the status of the intern and of the supervisor. Letters of agreement should be on file at the agency, and supervisors and interns should keep copies of all such contracts. Whether you are an intern or a supervisor, you will save yourself time and trouble by contacting the appropriate agencies rather than developing your own agreement letter. Sometimes very specific language is required in Letters of Agreement between clinics, interns, and supervisors. Check first with your professional organization and state licensing board before writing your own letters.

The two forms that follow, Employment Notification for Marriage, Family, and Child Counselor trainees, and Weekly Summary of Hours of Experience (accompanied by a Letter of Agreement), are produced by the California Department of Consumer Affairs. These forms relate to information that must be collected by interns; they help both you and the intern by ensuring that you are doing the proper paperwork (in this case, necessary for licensure in the state of California). These forms were

Employment Notification for Marriage, Fam~~ily~~ and Child Counselor Registered Interns

SAMPLE

Department of Consumer Affairs
BOARD OF BEHAVIORAL SCIENCE EXAMINERS
400 Q Street, Suite 1230
Yourville, US 00000-0000
Telephone (222) 555-6262

Business and Professions Code Section 4980.45 requires this information to be submitted to the board by the intern within 30 days of commencing employment or terminating employment **regardless of the employment setting.**

This is to notify the Board of Behavioral Science Examiners that as of ____1-2-94____
(date)

I ____Juan Castillo____ , MFCC Trainee,
(your name)

☑ became employed by ____Pacific Coast Counseling Center____
(name of organization)

☐ terminated employment at _____
(name of organization)

Type of Setting: (please check one)
☐ Private Practice
☐ Governmental Agency
☑ Nonprofit and Charitable Corporation
☐ Licensed Health Facility
☐ School, College, or University

These are the only acceptable settings for the accumulation of hours of experience.

Employer's Address ____123 Graff Blvd., Los Angeles, CA 90024____
(street)   (city)   (state, zip)

Employer's Telephone (213) 555-2012

Name of Supervisor (if different from employer) _____

My employer (supervisor if different than employer) holds the following license, which is current and in good standing:

	(license #)	(issue date)
Marriage, Family, and Child Counselor	NA 7421	MAY 1978
Clinical Social Worker		
Clinical Psychologist		
Psychiatrist (In accordance with Business and Professions Code Section 4980.45)		

I certify under the penalty of perjury under the laws of the State of California that the foregoing is true and correct.

____1-2-94____   *George R. Jones*   GEORGE R. JONES
(date)   (signature)   (print name)

Your daytime telephone number (213) 555-7927

NOTE: NOTIFICATION OF EMPLOYMENT OR TERMINATION OF EMPLOYMENT MUST BE RECEIVED, IN WRITING, WITHIN THIRTY (30) DAYS OF THE EMPLOYMENT OR TERMINATION DATE.

Letter of Agreement[1]
for Intern Supervision

SAMPLE

It is hereby agreed that *GEORGE R. JONES*
(supervisor)
hereinafter referred to as Supervisor, agrees to supervise the intern/trainee
listed below, for *PACIFIC COAST COUNSELING CENTER* .
(employer / organization)
Supervisor agrees to provide this service to *PACIFIC COAST COUNSELING CENTER*
(organization)
on a voluntary basis.[2] *PACIFIC COAST COUNSELING CENTER*
(organization)
agrees to allow Supervisor to supervise the intern/trainee listed below.
Supervisor agrees to ensure that the extent, kind, and quality of
counseling/psychotherapy performed by the intern/trainee listed below is
consistent with the intern's/trainee's training, education, and experience and is
appropriate in extent, kind, and quality. Supervisor agrees to ensure that the
counseling/psychotherapy performed by the intern/trainee listed below, and
the supervision provided by the supervisor, will be in accordance with
Chapter 13, Division 2 of the Business and Professions Code (the MFCC
Licensure Law) and any regulations promulgated thereunder.

The intern/trainee listed below is employed by *PACIFIC COAST COUNSELING CENTER*
(organization)
and performs counseling/psychotherapy services of a nature specified on
Chapter 13, Division 2 of the Business and Professions Code and any
regulations promulgated thereunder.

JUAN CASTILLO
Intern/Trainee (print)

Juan Castillo
Intern/Trainee (signature)

GEORGE R. JONES
Supervisor (print)

George R. Jones
Supervisor (signature)

PACIFIC COAST COUNSELING CENTER
Organization (print name)

123 GRAFF BLVD.
Street

LOS ANGELES, CA. 90024
City / State / Zip

LATICIA COLLINS, EXECUTIVE DIRECTOR
Authorized representative (print name and title)

29 Sept. 94
Dated

Laticia Collins
Authorized representative (signature)

(1) This letter of Agreement is to be signed and dated prior to providing services which are
to be counted as hours of experience.
(2) Although supervisor provides service to organization on a voluntary basis, intern or
trainee may pay supervisor for supervision.

WEEKLY SUMMARY OF HOURS OF EXPERIENCE   Year 19 _94_

(use a separate log for each supervised work setting and for each work status indicated below)

Name of MFCC Intern/Trainee _JUAN CASTILLO, MA_   BBSE file (if known) _3456_

Work Setting (name & address of employer) _PACIFIC COUNSELING CENTER, Los Angeles, CA_

Date Admitted to the Graduate Degree Program _1992_

Indicate the status of the MFCC Intern/Trainee for the hours logged:

Trainee in Practicum
(Registered: Yes No)

Post-Degree with Application Pending for Intern
Registration [B&P Code Section 4980.43(e)]

Trainee Not in Practicum
(Registered: Yes No)

✔ Registered Intern (MFCC Intern No. _NA7421_   )

Week of:	$^{10}/_3$	$^{10}/_{10}$	$^{10}/_{17}$	$^{10}/_{24}$								Total Hours
Couples, Family or Child Counseling, Psychotherapy (performed by you)	4	4	4	4								16
Individual Counseling or Psychotherapy (performed by you)	12	12	12	12								48
Group Therapy or Counseling (performed by you)												
Telephone Counseling (actual counseling time performed by you)	1	1	1	1								4
Supervision Individual Face-to-Face	1	1	1	1								4
Supervision Group	2	2	2	2								8
Workshops, Seminars, Training Sessions or Conferences	6	4	2	2								14
Admin. & Evaluating Psych. Test, Writing	2	2	2	2								8
Total per Week	28	26	24	24								102
Supervisor's Signature	*George R. Jones*	*George R. Jones*	*George R. Jones*	*George R. Jones*								

Form FPP-6-1/1-rev2/94 ©1994 GMS. Do not reproduce. For orders call (510) 865-5282, fax (510) 865-4295.

printed in *The California Therapist*, the journal of the California Association of Marriage and Family Therapists.

Different states and different licensing boards have different specific forms, but the concept is the same. In addition to whatever the state and your professional association offer, these forms can be obtained from the state consumer affairs agency and other sources. Due to obvious differences in state regulations, the actual forms or pamphlets you will need to conduct your private practice cannot be provided here.

Whether you are an intern or have been practicing for 20 years, call your state association on a yearly basis to check on the existence of forms, pamphlets, and hand-outs that may save you a great deal of time and money. Doing so will remove the possibility that you may be practicing (without your knowledge) illegally, unethically, or with outdated information.

Finally, ask the same question of these agencies that I ask new clients during the initial intake interview: "Is there anything I have not asked that is important for me to know?"

2

When the Client Arrives
Forms to be Used
in the Waiting Room

The forms in this chapter are those I place in a packet in my waiting room to inform potential patients about my credentials, their rights and responsibilities, and my rights and responsibilities.

For the individual patient, the packet will not include Guidelines for the Cliient Entering Group Therapy. Also, depending on your theoretical orientation, you may wish to operate as a tabula rasa (blank slate) and choose to leave out your curriculum vitae or biography.

Confidential Patient Information
For maintaining client records

As part of your initial phone contact, ask the patient to bring to the first session any information necessary for filling out insurance forms. In addition, ask the patient to write out a list of current medications, medical problems, and clinicians he or she may be seeing.

Since I use a 50-minute session beginning at 10 minutes after the hour, I ask patients to show up 10 minutes early to fill out the Confidential Client Information form. Along with this form, I include the Limits of Confidentiality form (to be signed by the patient), the Client's Bill of Rights, and a copy of my curriculum vitae.

I place all of these forms in a folder and, at times when I do not have a receptionist, I place the folder on a clipboard with a pencil. I attach a brief note to the folder asking the patient to please fill out and sign the forms. (I never write the patient's name on this note; instead, I use initials.) Prior to the appointment, I fill in the amount charged and the time limits of my consultation, and leave the folder in the waiting room.

I use a coding system for my patient's records. Here is a sample of one such code: 94-GOL-01. The first two numbers indicate the year of the beginning of treatment, the three letters are the first three letters of the patient's last name, and the last two numbers are assigned in case I have more than one patient with the same three letters. Michelle Silver's coding, as you will notice on all forms, is: 92-SIL-01.

CONFIDENTIAL CLIENT INFORMATION (page 1 of 2)

Welcome to my practice. Please fill out the following questions as completely as possible.
PLEASE PRINT OR WRITE LEGIBLY.

Client's Name	(Ms.) Mrs. Mr.	Silver _Last_	Michelle _First_	_Middle_	Marital Status: ☑ Single ☐ Married ☐ Separated ☐ Divorced ☐ Widowed ☐ Other

Client's Address	Street: 1234 Lands End Ave				
	City: Santa Monica	State: CA		Zip code: 90404	

Phone	Home: (213) 555-4321	Work: (213) 555-13-91	
	Age: 34	Birthdate: 9-21-58	Birthplace: Portland, OR

Education	No. of years: 14	Degree: AA	Field: Accounting
	Religious background: Roman Catholic	Current religion: None	

Spouse	Name: N/A	Age:	Occupation:	Years Married:

Children	M F Name:	Age:	M F Name:	Age:	M F Name:	Age:

Were you raised by: Both parents? **Yes**   Single parent?   Relative?   Other?

Father's name: **Anthony**   Age: **75**   Occupation: **Bus driver**

Mother's Name: **Mary**   Age: **65**   Occupation: **Homemaker**

Brothers and sisters (including yourself) in birth order:	Name: Maria Age: 46	Name: Tony, 44 Joe Age: 39
Name: Anna, 38	Frank, dead Age:	Name: Rob, 36 Michelle Age: 34	Name: Paul Age: 30

In your family was there a history of: ☑ Alcoholism?   ☐ Substance abuse?   ☐ Mental illness?
☐ Prolonged physical illness? What kind?

Current medications:

Significant medical problems: Gall Bladder Surgery, age 22
Foot Surgery, age 25

Have you had previous psychiatric care and/or counseling?   ☐ Yes   ☑ No
If yes, give: Name of clinician   Degree/License   Sessions from   to

Have you ever been hospitalized for substance abuse, alcoholism, eating disorders, or other psychiatric disorders?
☐ Yes   ☑ No   Details:

CONFIDENTIAL CLIENT INFORMATION (page 2 of 2)

Client or Guardian employed by: **E † M Computer Corporation**

Employer's address: **806 Claret Ave**

City: **Los Angeles**   State: **CA**   Zip: **90066** Phone (**213**) **555 - 1234**

Name of insurance company: **National Insurance Co** Name of insured: **Michelle Silver**

Group No. **MED 3218234**   Member No. **28147**

Driver's License No. **KZ999**   Social Security No. **222-22-2222**

Insurance company billing address: **2780 Central Blvd.**

City: **Los Angeles**   State: **CA**   Zip: **90066** Phone (**213**) **555 - 1212**

Spouse employed by:

Employer's address:

City: State: Zip: Phone ( )

Name of insurance company: Name of insured:

Group No.   Member No.

Driver's License No.   Social Security No.

Insurance company billing address:

City: State: Zip: Phone ( )

I, **Michelle Silver** , understand and agree to pay **George Jones, Ph.D.** the amount of
(Person responsible for payment) (Clinician's name)
$ **90.00** at the conclusion of each **50** -minute consultation.

I understand that I am responsible for payment for consultations not cancelled 24 hours in advance. Payment for services is rendered at the conclusion of the consultation unless other arrangements have been made. I hereby authorize the clinician to furnish information to insurance carriers concerning my treatment. I understand that I am responsible for all payments. Any monies received by the clinician from the above insurance companies over and above my indebtedness will be refunded to me when my bill is paid in full.

Client's Signature: **Michelle Silver** Date: **April 21, 1992**

Spouse's Signature: Date:

Parent/Guardian's Signature: Date:

> I will be happy to discuss my fees, schedule of payments, or any
> other questions relating to billing or insurance.
> Please do not hesitate to ask.

Limits of Confidentiality
For detailing limits of confidentiality

The following limits of confidentiality, as outlined on the forms, are currently practiced in the state of California. Research has shown that the California standards of practice are among the most stringent in the United States. Thus they are used as an example. I include the Limits of Confidentiality (even though informed consent is not required in California) because I believe it is ethical to inform a perspective client that limits to confidentiality do exist, and that a good client relationship is based on full disclosure on both sides.

The second Limits of Confidentiality form is to be used by interns and trainees. It is professionally ethical—and in many states a legal requirement—that clients be informed that they are being counseled by an intern under supervision. An intern is legally obligated to disclose all information about clients to the supervisor. In California, this notification must be given in writing before counseling begins.

The opposing view on informed consent holds that signing this form will lead a client to withhold important information that must be reported for the health and safety of others, such as child abuse and elder abuse.

Limits of Confidentiality

Information discussed in the therapy setting is held confidential and will not be shared without written permission except under the following conditions:

1. The client threatens suicide.

2. The client threatens harm to another person(s), including murder, assault, or other physical harm.

3. The client is a minor (under 18) and reports suspected child abuse, including but not limited to, physical beatings, and sexual abuse.

4. The client reports abuse of the elderly.

5. The client reports sexual exploitation by a therapist.

State law mandates that mental health professionals may need to report these situations to the appropriate persons and/or agencies.

Communications between the clinician and client will otherwise be deemed confidential as stated under the laws of this state.

Having read and understood the above, I agree to these limits of confidentiality.

MICHELLE SILVER   9-26-92
_____   _____
Name of Client or Guardian   Date

Michelle Silver
_____
Signature of Client or Guardian

George R Jones, Ph.D.
_____
Signature of Clinician

Form FPP-9-1/1-rev2/94 ©1994 GMS. Limited permission to photocopy only. For orders call (510) 865-5282, fax (510) 865-4295.

Limits of Confidentiality
Intern/Trainee

Information discussed in the therapy setting is held confidential and will not be shared without written permission except under the following conditions:

1. The client threatens suicide.

2. The client threatens harm to another person(s), including murder, assault, or other physical harm.

3. The client is a minor (under 18) and reports suspected child abuse, including but not limited to, physical beatings, and sexual abuse.

4. The client reports abuse of the elderly.

5. The client reports sexual exploitation by a therapist.

State law mandates that mental health professionals may need to report these situations to the appropriate persons and/or agencies.

Further, as a registered intern/trainee who is under the supervision of a licensed practitioner, therapy sessions will be discussed with a supervisor or professional colleagues as deemed necessary.

Communications between the clinician and client will otherwise be deemed confidential as stated under the laws of this state.

Having read and understood the above, I agree to these limits of confidentiality.

MICHELLE SILVER
_____
Name of Client or Guardian

Michelle Silver
_____
Signature of Client or Guardian

9-26-92
_____
Date

Juan Castillo
_____
Signature of Intern/Trainee

George R. Jones, Ph.D.
_____
Signature of Supervisor

Form FPP-10-1/1-rev2/94 ©1994 GMS. Limited permission to photocopy only. For orders call (510) 865-5282, fax (510) 865-4295.

Client's Bill of Rights
For itemizing client's rights

The Client's Bill of Rights and the group therapy guidelines that follow are forms for my client's information only, they do not need to be signed. Which one you use will depend on whether you are seeing a client individually or in a group. Some states require or will be requiring the clinician to post, hand out, or have prospective clients sign, forms or booklets on ethical and unethical practices, and inform the client where he or she can report breaches of ethics (covered in the discussion of ethical standards later in this chapter). State and local associations, as well as the state licensing board, will give you this information.

Client's Bill of Rights

You, the client, have the right to:

- receive respectful treatment that will be helpful to you

- receive a particular type of treatment or end treatment without obligation or harassment

- a safe environment, free from sexual, physical, and emotional abuse

- report unethical and illegal behavior by a therapist

- ask questions about your therapy

- request and receive full information about the therapist's professional capabilities, including licensure, education, training, experience, professional association membership, specialization, and limitations

- have written information about fees, methods of payment, insurance reimbursement, number of sessions, substitutions (in cases of vacation and emergencies), and cancellation policies *before* beginning therapy

- refuse electronic recording, but you may request it if you wish

- refuse to answer any questions or disclose any information you choose not to reveal

- know the limits of confidentiality and the circumstances in which a therapist is legally required to disclose information to others

- know if there are supervisors, consultants, students, or others with whom your therapist will discuss your case

- request, and in most cases receive, a summary of your file, including the diagnosis, your progress, and type of treatment

- request the transfer of a copy of your file to any therapist or agency you choose

- receive a second opinion at any time about your therapy or therapist's methods

- request that the therapist inform you of your progress

Guidelines for the Client Entering Group Therapy
For orienting new clients entering a group

The following guidelines were written by a colleague who runs a private practice. This form is an excellent example of the way a clinician can introduce a new client into the private practice. You may wish to prepare similar guidelines and protocols to encourage client cooperation and to serve as guidelines for clients to give to family members, significant others, and other acquaintances who might be considering (in this case) group therapy.

Guidelines used this way will not only aid you in delivering your services to a more receptive clientele, but can be used as handouts for speaking engagements. These guidelines (which you are free to use) also help clarify clinical goals and objectives. At the same time, they may encourage appropriate prospective clients and discourage inappropriate prospects.

Guidelines for the Client Entering Group Therapy
(page 1 of 2)

Therapy Groups are based on the assumption that much of the behavior we have learned may block communication, get in the way of creative relationships, and interfere with intimacy and warmth with others, especially friends, associates, and family. The following suggestions may help those attending groups become more open, and able to give and receive clear communication with others.

1. **Speak in the first person.** Use "I." Instead of saying "people feel" or "you get the feeling . . . " etc., say, "I think . . . " or "I feel . . . ". This gives more of the flavor of *you* rather than broad generalities.

2. **Speak directly to individuals.** Look at people's faces and speak directly to them. If another person asks you: "How do you feel about Bill right now?" for example, turn to Bill and say: "Bill, I feel you were very kind to me a minute ago when you said . . . " or "I resent you right now," or whatever—rather than facing the person who asked you the question originally.

3. **Speak from your honest feelings and thoughts.** There is no taboo on language, thoughts, or expressions in this kind of group. Failing to communicate exactly what you feel—whether it is anger or affection or indifference toward another—is considered "kindness" by the world. Yet it is often the cruelest thing we can do to someone else. It is based on lying, on not trusting the other's ability to handle our honest feelings. How can people respond properly if they have never been honestly told how others feel about and react to them?

4. **Be aware of your thoughts and feelings in the moment.** Express them at the earliest appropriate time. Be aware, even if you cannot express your perception of that moment. We cannot live creatively if we cloud the present with the imagined past or a dreamed-of future that never comes. We freely live only in one dimension of time—the here and now.

5. **Read the messages from your own body.** Your body is a most basic, tangible aspect of you. It is continually giving you messages. The open or closed position of your limbs, sweating palms, feeling "fidgety," rapid heartbeat, moving to a closer or more remote seat, blushing, increased elimination needs—all these may be telling you that you are excited, anxious, angry, worried, embarrassed, wanting to be closer to a person, aroused, etc. Noticing these messages helps you to keep in touch with yourself.

6. **Be as spontaneous as possible.** Too often we mull things over, choose careful language, wait too long, try to be polite, wait our turn to speak or react. This can water down or negate our freshness, sparkle, and genuineness. Try to let ideas, thoughts, and feelings spill out and over as they come; they will convey the true "you."

7. **Report "side conversations" to the main group.** If, during a break, a meal, or between sessions you hold a side conversation with anyone in which you comment on the group, the interaction, or a person, you should report the feelings expressed back to the group or persons. The idea here is to speak face-to-face and keep feelings out in the open.

8. **Be aware of the roles you take and your characteristic behavior.** We tend to behave similarly in many situations. For instance, some of us tend to be ready to argue and challenge. Others tend to withdraw or run away from a confrontation, while others are "peacemakers" or compromisers. Some people tend to behave differently in each situation, carefully sampling

Guidelines for the Client Entering Group Therapy
(page 2 of 2)

the popular opinion and then trying to conform to it. Sometimes we behave in an therapy group much as we do with our mate, friends, parents, associates, or in other groups. By observing yourself and others in this group you come to helpful insights.

9. **Be aware of how persons in this group remind you of other significant people in your past or present life.** For instance, a certain woman may remind you of your mother, wife, or an old girlfriend. A certain man may remind you of your father, boss, or rival. Interacting with those persons can often work out old problems, affections, hurts, joys, and sorrows even if the person is not completely like the person she or he reminds you of.

10. **Listen actively.** Good communication involves not only clear expression of what you think and feel, but also listening clearly to the words, feelings, and behavior communications of others. (It is good to attempt to occasionally "crawl into another's skin" or "wear his moccasins" in your imagination in order to understand him or her.) Most of us have a tendency to read in things *we* feel or agree with while missing what the person is trying to convey. We also tend to "read out" or ignore things a person is expressing that bother us for some reason. Techniques such as repeating back to a person what you *thought* he or she said *before* you answer may be helpful if it does not dampen spontaneity. In this way one can learn to allow for one's biases and prejudices which may distort what is going on in and around us.

11. **Don't speak for others.** This involves using phrases like: "most men think . . . ," "a woman always feels . . . ," "I think Bill feels you don't like him . . . ," etc. Speak for yourself, or *ask* the person—or everyone present—what she or he or they are feeling or thinking. If you feel empathy for a person, or feel like defending or attacking someone, describe what you are experiencing at that moment rather than attributing it to others or putting your own feelings off onto someone else.

12. **Try to have genuine "encounters" with others.** The aim of an encounter is not necessarily to fight, or to avoid anger, or to always be on good terms with everyone or to "love" everyone. It is rather to realize that the basic stuff of life is to contact, interact, feel, and communicate meaningfully with others. A quarrel is often better than ignoring someone else. To know that you have been true to yourself while meaningfully interacting with another who is also being true to herself or himself is a major aim of such group experiences. It can also have favorable effects on your social relationships after the group ends.

13. **Expect periods of silence.** Although they may seem, at first, uncomfortable, creative things can occur in our awareness and consciousness. Use silence to become aware of what is happening to you and within you.

14. **Post-therapy group feelings, awarenesses, and anxieties are normal.** Know that follow-up appointments with the therapist-counselor-leader are available and often desirable.

Curriculum Vitae and Biography
For details regarding the therapist's credentials

A sample of a curriculum vitae (CV) and a biography are on the following pages. Several years ago there was talk among the legislature in California about requiring professionals to give a CV to all new clients. To my knowledge it got lost in the shuffle.

I have always included a copy of my CV and biography in the initial interview packet. Those of you who practice using analytic orthodoxy may not wish to do so, but I believe that all practitioners should give to their clients, or have available, their CV or abbreviated biography.

A biography can be inserted in workshop booklets and included in handouts to attendees of lectures and speaking engagements.

Curriculum Vitae

SAMPLE

MICHAEL I. GOLD, PH.D.
1234 W. Main Blvd., Suite 5, Los Angeles, CA 90000
(310) 555-1212, (213) 555-1212

EDUCATION

1961 Santa Monica City College, A.A., Fine Arts/English
1963 UCLA, B.A., Fine Arts/Anthropology
1964 UCLA, M.S., Fine Arts/Education
1969 California State University, Northridge, M.A., Psychological Foundations: Counseling
1981 Columbia Pacific University, Ph.D., Clinical Psychology
      Dissertation: The Design and Implementation of an Intern Training Program
      for the South Central Free Clinic

CREDENTIALS

California: General Secondary—ZZ123456
California: Standard Secondary—12345XY
California: Standard Junior College—123ABC
California: General Service/Pupil Personnel—XX12345
California: General Service/Administrative—YY1234
California: Community College Student Personnel Worker—98765
California: Community College Counseling—87654
California: Licensed Marriage, Family and Child Counselor XY123456

EMPLOYMENT HISTORY—EDUCATION

1965–1989 Centinela Valley Union High School District
           12227 Hawthorne Way, Hawthorne, CA 90250
           Classroom Instructor
           Subjects taught: English, Speech, Psychology, American Government, World Studies,
               Consumer Education, Remedial Reading, World History, Drama, Sociology,
               Substance Abuse, Film as Literature
           School Counselor
           School Assistant Principal
           School Principal

1971   Pepperdine University
           Subject: Teacher Training—Behavioral Paradigm

1983–Present: Antioch University
           Subjects taught: Psychopathology, Advanced Psychopathology, Existential
           Psychotherapy, Oral Case Presentation

CLINICAL EXPERIENCE

1968–1971 Los Angeles Free Clinic, Psychological Intern

1971–1972 Neuropsychiatric Institute—UCLA, Occupational Therapy
           Supervisors:
           Lars Hambrook, Ph.D., L.A. Free Clinic
           Leslie Pain, L.A. Free Clinic
           Sigmund Helms, M.D.—N.P.I., UCLA
           Richard Hasstle, M.D.—N.P.I., UCLA
           Henry Roosman, M.A.—Private Practice
           Manfred Brooke, M.A.—Private Practice

Joshua Crane, Ph.D.—Private Practice: Hypnosis
Ignace Mercer, M.D.—Private Practice
Jeffrey Just, Ph.D.—Private Practice

1968–Present: Private Practice, Licensed Psychotherapist:
    MFCC XY 12345 Los Angeles and Manhattan Beach offices

COMMUNITY PRACTICE

1968–1971 Los Angeles Free Clinic, Psychological Intern
1980–1985 Clinical Director: Psychology Department, South Bay Free Clinic

AFFILIATIONS

American Psychological Association—Division Five
California Association of Marriage and Family Therapists
California Teachers Association
American Civil Liberties Union
Performing Member: Society for the Magical Arts
Professional Member: Society for the Preservation of the Variety Arts
American Federation of Television and Radio Artists
Screen Actor's Guild

HONORS

Dean's List—UCLA
Who's Who in California
Outstanding School Administrator—Los Angeles County School System
Honorary Chairman—South Bay Patrons Association

PUBLICATIONS

Environmental Qualities Magazine: "The Socialization of Marijuana," "Frankenstein Meets the Feminist Movement"

South Bay Magazine: "Group Sex: An Analysis of Swinging," "Are You a Homosexual?" "Psyche-Paths"—a monthly reader response column

Medical Aspects of Human Sexuality: "Using Patient Humor to Uncover Hidden Psychopathology"

EDUCATIONAL TELEVISION

Wrote and produced teacher-training films for the Department of Health, Education and Welfare under the direction of Jesse Helms—UCLA: *Assertive Discipline, Analogous Practice,* and *Testing.*

MEDIA CONSULTATIONS

Technical Consultant to television writers, directors, and actors of *R*I*O*T, After R*I*O*T, St. Somewhere, Bitters,* ABC'S *Wide World of Entertainment,* RKO's *The Horror Shop,* ABC's *3-3-0,* Fox Television's *Henry Trick Show, David Moster, Everything in Common, Moss Dreams.*

CURRENTLY

Private Practice: Manhattan Beach and Los Angeles
Instructor: Antioch Graduate Psychology Program
Consultation: Hotel 6 (Employee Relations)

HOBBIES AND AVOCATIONS

Guitar, certified SCUBA diver/instructor, close-up magician, Hawaiian stamp collector, videotaping family histories, screen and stage writing, collector of rare documents, extensive travel

Biography

MICHAEL I. GOLD, PH.D.
1234 W. Main Blvd, Suite 5, Los Angeles, CA 90000
(310) 555-1212, (213) 555-1212

Dr. Gold was born June 19, 1942 in Chicago, Illinois, and moved to Los Angeles at age ten. He holds advanced degrees in the Fine Arts and Psychology. Dr. Gold has been practicing psychotherapy in Los Angeles and Manhattan Beach for twenty-three years. He also teaches Psychopathology, Clinical Case Presentation, and Existential Psychology in the Graduate Program at Antioch University.

Dr. Gold has served as technical consultant for motion pictures and television. His credits include *R*I*O*T, After R*I*O*T, So-So Crimes, Married White Female, Moss Dreams, St. Somewhere,* and *Bitters*. He is a regular consultant for the Reno, Tahoe Chamber of Commerce and Hotel 6 and Casino on issues of management/employee relations and guest/employee relations.

Dr. Gold is presently writing several books for publication, including *When Somebody You Love Is in Therapy, Fundamentals of a Private Practice,* and *Oral Case Presentation*. He is also developing a seminar entitled "Magic in Nursing," a technique of teaching magic to hospital patients in order to accelerate their recovery and boost morale.

Dr. Gold is single and lives alone with his cat, Tigger. He is a performing magician and member at The Magic Castle in Los Angeles. He claims that his daughter, Julie, is crazy about him.

Ethical Standards
For complaints of violations of ethical standards

The following samples are taken from booklets printed by state licensing agencies and state and national associations. Your licensing agency or association may have booklets or guidelines that they are willing to give for free, have you reproduce at your own expense, or pay for at very reasonable fees. Some of these booklets concern the ethics of our profession, some concern legalities related to our work, some are directed to the psychotherapist, and others are directed toward your patient population. These last can be placed on your waiting room table or given to each of your clients.

With the permission of the following state and national associations, portions of various pamphlets are reproduced here. These were obtained from the American Psychological Association, the American Psychiatric Association, and the American Association of Marriage and Family Therapy. For complete booklets, write to your state or national association.

Ethical Principles of Psychologists of the American Psychological Association

Principle 1: Responsibility
In providing services, psychologists maintain the highest standards of their profession. They accept responsibility for the consequences of their acts and make every effort to ensure that their services are used appropriately.

Principle 2: Competence
The maintenance of high standards of competence is a responsibility shared by all psychologists in the interest of the public and the profession as a whole. Psychologists recognize the boundaries of their competence and the limitations of their techniques. They only provide services and only use techniques for which they are qualified by training and experience. In those areas in which recognized standards do not yet exist, psychologists take whatever precautions are necessary to protect the welfare of their clients. They maintain knowledge of current scientific and professional information related to the services they render.

Principle 3: Moral and Legal Standards
Psychologists' moral and ethical standards of behavior are a personal

matter to the same degree as they are for any other citizen, except as these may compromise the fulfillment of their professional responsibilities or reduce the public trust in psychology and psychologists. Regarding their own behavior, psychologists are sensitive to prevailing community standards and to the possible impact that conformity to or deviation from these standards may have upon the quality of their performance as psychologists. Psychologists are also aware of the possible impact of their public behavior upon the ability of colleagues to perform their professional duties.

Principle 4: Public Statements
Public statements, announcements of services, advertising, and promotional activities of psychologists serve the purpose of helping the public make informed judgments and choices. Psychologists represent accurately and objectively their professional qualifications, affiliations, and functions, as well as those of the institutions or organizations with which they or the statements may be associated. In public statements providing psychological information or professional opinions or providing information about the availability of psychological products, publications, and services, psychologists base their statements on scientifically acceptable psychological findings and techniques with full recognition of the limits and uncertainties of such evidence.

Principle 5: Confidentiality
Psychologists have a primary obligation to respect the confidentiality of information obtained from persons in the course of their work as psychologists. They reveal such information to others only with the consent of the person or the person's legal representative, except in the unusual circumstances in which not to do so would result in clear danger to the person or to others. Where appropriate, psychologists inform their clients of the legal limits of confidentiality.

Principle 6: Welfare of the Consumer
Psychologists respect the integrity and protect the welfare of the people and groups with whom they work. When conflicts of interest arise between clients and psychologists' employing institutions, psychologists clarify the nature and direction of their loyalties and responsibilities and keep all parties informed of their commitments. Psychologists fully inform consumers as to the purpose and nature of an evaluative, treatment, educational, or training procedure, and they freely acknowledge that clients, students, or participants in research have freedom of choice with regard to participation.

Principle 7: Professional Relationships
Psychologists act with due regard for the needs, special competencies, and obligations of their colleagues in psychology and other professions. They respect the prerogatives and obligations of the institutions or organizations with which these other colleagues are associated.

Principle 8: Assessment Techniques
In the development, publication, and utilization of psychological assessment techniques, psychologists make every effort to promote the welfare and best interests of the client. They guard against the misuse of assessment results. They respect the client's right to know the results, the interpretations made, and the bases for their conclusions and recommendations. Psychologists make every effort to maintain the security of tests and other assessment techniques within the limits of legal mandates. They strive to ensure the appropriate use of assessment techniques by others.

Principle 9: Research with Human Participants
The decision to undertake research rests upon a considered judgment by the individual psychologist about how best to contribute to psychological science and human welfare. Having made the decision to conduct research, the psychologist considers alternative directions in which research energies and resources might be invested. On the basis of this consideration, the psychologist carries out the investigation with respect and concern for the dignity and welfare of the people who participate and with cognizance of federal and state regulations and professional standards governing the conduct of research with human participants.

Principle 10: Care and Use of Animals
An investigator of animal behavior strives to advance understanding of basic behavioral principles and/or to contribute to the improvement of human health and welfare. In seeking these ends, the investigator ensures the welfare of animals and treats them humanely. Laws and regulations notwithstanding, an animal's immediate protection depends upon the scientist's own conscience.

Reprinted with permission from American Psychologist *(March 1990, pp. 390–395).*

Code of Ethics of the American Association for Marriage and Family Therapy

1. Responsibility to Clients
Marriage and family therapists advance the welfare of families and individuals. They respect the rights of those persons seeking their assistance, and make reasonable efforts to ensure that their services are used appropriately.

2. Confidentiality
Marriage and family therapists have unique confidentiality concerns because the client in a therapeutic relationship may be more than one person. Therapists respect and guard confidences of each individual client.

3. Professional Competence and Integrity
Marriage and family therapists maintain high standards of professional competence and integrity.

4. Responsibility to Students, Employees, and Supervisees
Marriage and family therapists do not exploit the trust and dependency of students, employees, and supervisees.

5. Responsibility to Research Participants
Investigators respect the dignity and protect the welfare of participants in research and are aware of federal and state laws and regulations and professional standards governing the conduct of research.

6. Responsibility to the Profession
Marriage and family therapists respect the rights and responsibilities of professional colleagues and participate in activities which advance the goals of the profession.

7. Financial Arrangements
Marriage and family therapists make financial arrangements with clients, third party payors, and supervisees that are reasonably understandable and conform to accepted professional practices.

8. Advertising
Marriage and family therapists engage in appropriate informational activities, including those that enable laypersons to choose professional services on an informed basis.

Reprinted with permission from the American Association for Marriage and Family Therapy.

Principles of Medical Ethics of the American Psychiatric Association

Preamble

The medical profession has long subscribed to a body of ethical statements developed primarily for the benefit of the patient. As a member of this profession, a physician must recognize responsibility not only to patients but also to society, to other health professionals, and to self. The following Principles, adopted by the American Psychiatric Association, are not laws but standards of conduct, which define the essentials of honorable behavior for the physician.

Section 1

A physician shall be dedicated to providing competent medical service with compassion and respect for human dignity.

Section 2

A physician shall deal honestly with patients and colleagues, and strive to expose those physicians deficient in character or competence, or who engage in fraud or deception.

Section 3

A physician shall respect the law and also recognize a responsibility to seek changes in those requirements which are contrary to the best interests of the patient.

Section 4

A physician shall respect the rights of patients, of colleagues, and of other health professionals, and shall safeguard patient confidences within the constraints of the law.

Section 5

A physician shall continue to study, apply, and advance scientific knowledge, make relevant information available to patients, colleagues, and the public, obtain consultation, and use the talents of other health professionals when indicated.

Section 6

A physician shall, in the provision of appropriate patient care, except in emergencies, be free to choose whom to serve, with whom to associate, and the environment in which to provide medical services.

Section 7
A physician shall recognize a responsibility to participate in activities contributing to an improved community.

Reprinted with permission from the American Psychiatric Association.

3

When the Client Is in Session
Forms to Be Used During the Initial Intake Session

The forms in this chapter are fundamental to practitioners of any theoretical school. These forms will be necessary to use with all patients, especially for legal purposes. Whether you collect your fee at the beginning or end of the session, billing statements and billing records must be available for IRS audit. Most states that license psychotherapists have legal precedents that require the clinician to keep some form of notations relating to patients. In the course of your practice, you will experience the necessity to present these forms, or a summary of their contents.

Clinical Notations
For the therapist's record of a client's session

The Clinical Notations form is probably the most significant form you will fill out during the course of your practice. It is a document that can be admitted as evidence for or against your client in a court of law.

I once counseled a client who became involved in a lawsuit. Without being notified by my client or my client's attorney, I was served a subpoena *duces tecum* ("you are summoned to bring the things") for the upcoming case. Upon contacting my client and—with his written release—his attorney, I found out that my client unwittingly gave up his right to confidentiality. He had sued another individual, and in the suit his attorney had stated that they may be suing for "emotional pain and suffering." In such cases, the therapist may not have the right, based on state codes of evidence, to withhold notations or withhold giving a deposition.

Now, I let my clients know in advance that if they are going to be involved in any legal action, they should inform me and give me permission in writing to speak to their representatives about matters of confidentiality as related to the field of psychotherapy and the laws of the state.

The standard of practice for clinical notations can be remembered with the acronym SOAP: "S"—for something that the client *says*; "O"—for something the clinician *observes*; "A"—for the client's *affect* during the consultation; "P"—for any *prescriptions*, medical or verbal, that you have given.

When writing clinical notations covering these four areas, keep in mind that years later these records may be subpoenaed or become a matter of record for a state investigating agency. For example, a member of the Treasury Department may present you with an authorization for release of records signed by a client you had treated long ago. He may be investigating her background for a security clearance in her new job.

Let's assume you were seeing this client 10 years ago. During a session, she discussed her sexual orientation. Let's further assume that, like most adolescents, she had a frightening dream containing manifest homosexual or bisexual content. At that point in her life she had never engaged in sexual behavior and was concerned that the dream meant she was gay. When making your notations, you could either write "discussed sexual orientation" or "discussed bisexuality and homosexuality." It is sad, but true, that a person's sexual orientation may exclude him or her from clearances or jobs, and such notations could be detrimental to a person's career.

As a professional, you must view your records not only in the context of your client's present situation, but also in light of how a notation made 10 years from now can affect a patient. This is especially true if these records will be left at a clinic without your direct supervision.

I cannot emphasize enough the term *professional judgment*. All facts, as well as judgments, are arguable. One of the reasons we are called *professionals* is that we must make judgments, minute by minute, for which there are no road maps.

Page No. *1*	**CLINICAL NOTATIONS**

Client's Name:	*MICHELLE*

Client's ID No.	*92-SIL-01*

Year:	*1992*

Date: *9/26* • Client's remarks • Therapist's observations • Client's affect • Recommendations & interventions	*TALKED ABOUT ACCIDENT.* *PT. GAINED WEIGHT.* *AFFECT: DEPRESSED — INTERMITTENT CRYING* *Rx: SUPPORTED AND AFFIRMED PAIN*
Date: *9/30* • Client's remarks • Therapist's observations • Client's affect • Recommendations & interventions	*"NOT SLEEPING"* *PT. PALE, DRAWN* *PT. MOROSE* *Rx: SUGGESTED PT. DO THINGS TO BE GOOD TO HERSELF AND TO REFLECT ON HOW SHE IS A WORTHY PERSON*
Date: *10/2* • Client's remarks • Therapist's observations • Client's affect • Recommendations & interventions	*"I GOT A FULL NIGHT'S SLEEP YESTERDAY."* *PT. MORE RESTED THAN LAST SESSION* *AFFECT: LOW-KEY, NON-DEPRESSED* *Rx: ASKED PATIENT TO REFLECT ON SIMILARITIES BETWEEN HER BOSS AND FEELINGS SHE HAD AS A CHILD AROUND AUTHORITY FIGURES.*
Date: • Client's remarks • Therapist's observations • Client's affect • Recommendations & interventions	

Mental Status Examination
For the establishment of a diagnosis

Mental status examinations are necessary for the establishment of a diagnosis. The following Mental Status Examination form can be filled out during or after the client interview.

After your initial intake interview, you may find that there are many gaps in the mental status examination. This form is designed to help you fill in the gaps. On more than one occasion I have treated a client who was so despondent or psychotic that I could not gather enough reliable information at the time. This form tells me both what I know and what I need to find out.

Another special aspect of this form is that it is designed for a client or a client and significant other. This allows the clinician to compare the mental status of two people in a conjoint session.

The mental status examination should be readministered once every three to six months so that you can gauge progress or deterioration in your client.

MENTAL STATUS EXAMINATION (page 1 of 4)

DATE: *9-26-92*   CLINICIAN: *GEORGE R. JONES*

CLIENT'S NAME: *92-SIL-01*   DAY PHONE: *(213) 555-1391*

SPOUSE'S NAME: NIGHT PHONE: *(213) 555-4321*

REFERRED BY: DATE:

	CLIENT	SPOUSE
PRESENTATION PROBLEM(S): *NOT SLEEPING WELL, DEPRESSION, IRRITATED, CAN'T CONCENTRATE, CRIES OFTEN*		
PRECIPITATING EVENT(S): *CAR ACCIDENT (8-26-92)*		
PRESENTATION SYMPTOM(S): *TIRED, LISTLESS, DEPRESSED*		
PRESENTATION SIGN(S): *SLUMPED POSTURE, TEARFUL, LOOKS TIRED, APPEARS IRRITABLE*		
OTHER:		

DSM-III-R	MULTIAXIAL DIAGNOSTIC ASSESSMENT	
AXIS I	Clinical Syndrome(s) *INSOMNIA DISORDER MAJOR DEPRESSION*	
AXIS II	Personality Disorder/ Developmental Disorder(s) *DEFERRED*	
AXIS III	Medical Disorder(s) *SEE MEDICAL AND PSYCHIATRIC REPORT*	
AXIS IV	Psychosocial Stressor (0-6) *4*	
AXIS V	(a) Highest level of current functioning *40*	
	(b) Highest level of functioning in the past year *50-60*	

Form FPP-15-1/4-rev2/94 ©1994 GMS. Limited permission to photocopy only. For orders call (510) 865-5282, fax (510) 865-4295.

Circle appropriate findings	MENTAL STATUS EXAMINATION (page 2 of 4)				
	CLIENT			**SPOUSE**	
I. APPEARANCE	actual age	⟨older⟩	younger	actual age	older	younger
Gender & Race:	FEMALE, CAU.					
Height: 5'8"	⟨tall⟩	medium	short	tall	medium	short
Build:	thin	⟨medium ⟷ heavy⟩		thin	medium	heavy
	athletic	very obese		athletic	very obese	
Pupils:	⟨equal⟩	constricted	dilated	equal	constricted	dilated
Hygienic state:	⟨clean⟩			clean		disheveled
	unshaven		odorous	unshaven		odorous
Clothing:	⟨neat⟩	untidy	peculiar	neat	untidy	peculiar
Posture:	⟨normal ⟷ slumped⟩		rigid	normal	slumped	rigid
Facial expression:	amiable	happy	⟨worried⟩	amiable	happy	worried
	⟨tense⟩	angry	suspicious	tense	angry	suspicious
	⟨sad⟩		immobile	sad		immobile
2. ATTITUDE & BEHAVIOR	⟨alert ⟷ confused⟩		drowsy	alert	confused	drowsy
	hypervigilant		stuporous	hypervigilant		stuporous
Attention span:	⟨satisfactory ⟷ poor⟩			satisfactory		poor
	distractable			distractable		
Eye contact:	good		stares into space	good		stares into space
	⟨avoidant⟩			avoidant		
Muscular movement:	normal	fidgety	⟨excited⟩	normal	fidgety	excited
	hyperactive	⟨hypoactive⟩		hyperactive	hypoactive	
Mannerisms:	⟨none⟩	pacing	handwringing	none	pacing	handwringing
	echopraxia	stereotypy	tics	echopraxia	stereotypy	tics
Physiological signs:	none	tearful	tremorous	none	tearful	tremorous
	⟨crying⟩	blushing	sweating	crying	blushing	sweating
Demeanor:	⟨friendly⟩	worried	boastful	friendly	worried	boastful
	⟨trustful⟩	demanding	⟨evasive⟩	trustful	demanding	evasive
	dramatic	covertly seductive		dramatic	covertly seductive	
	self-deprecatory	arrogant		self-deprecatory	arrogant	
	cold	irritable	apathetic	cold	irritable	apathetic
	⟨reserved⟩	resistive	hostile	reserved	resistive	hostile
	⟨cooperative⟩	uncooperative		cooperative	uncooperative	
3. MOOD	⟨anxious⟩	⟨fearful⟩	⟨suspicious⟩	anxious	fearful	suspicious
	⟨depressed⟩	euphoric	relaxed	depressed	euphoric	relaxed
	⟨angry⟩	guilty	ashamed	angry	guilty	ashamed
		indifferent			indifferent	
	(mild	moderate	severe)	(mild	moderate	severe)

Form FPP-15-2/4-rev2/94 ©1994 GMS. Limited permission to photocopy only. For orders call (510) 865-5282, fax (510) 865-4295.

Circle appropriate findings	MENTAL STATUS EXAMINATION (page 3 of 4)	
	CLIENT	SPOUSE
4. AFFECT	(appropriate to content) (labile) inappropriate blunted flat	appropriate to content labile inappropriate blunted flat
5. SPEECH	soft normal loud screaming	soft normal loud screaming
Mother tongue:	(English) Spanish Other	English Spanish Other
Quantity:	normal mute verbose answers only questions	normal mute verbose answers only questions
Speed:	(slow ←→ normal) rapid pressured	slow normal rapid pressured
Impediments:	(none) stutter lisp slur	none stutter lisp slur
Quality:	unremarkable flight of ideas (concrete ←→ circumstantial) joking overinclusive verbigeration neologistic echolalic precise senseless repetition tangential confabulating monotone obscenities	unremarkable flight of ideas concrete circumstantial joking overinclusive verbigeration neologistic echolalic precise senseless repetition tangential confabulating monotone obscenities
6. THOUGHT & ASSOCIATION	(logical ←→ blocking) loose incoherent clang (rhyming)	logical blocking loose incoherent clang (rhyming)
7. SOMATIC FUNCTIONING		
Appetite:	good (poor) unable to eat (weight loss) or gain in last _3_ months current weight: _135_	good poor unable to eat weight loss or gain in last ___ months current weight:
Sleep:	7–8 hours 9+ hours (5–7 hours) 4–5 hours less than 4 hours nightmares trouble going to sleep (early morning wakefulness)	7–8 hours 9+ hours 5–7 hours 4–5 hours less than 4 hours nightmares trouble going to sleep early morning wakefulness
Substance use:	amphetamines sedatives alcohol heroin speed (caffeine) nicotine marijuana cocaine PCP other: (mild (moderate) severe)	amphetamines sedatives alcohol heroin speed caffeine nicotine marijuana cocaine PCP other: (mild moderate severe)
Current medications:	*NONE*	
Medical problems:	*POSSIBLE INJURIES FROM AUTO ACCIDENT 8-26-92*	

Circle appropriate findings	MENTAL STATUS EXAMINATION (page 4 of 4)	
	CLIENT	SPOUSE
8. PROVERB RESPONSE		
Bird in the Hand	abstract (concrete) peculiar	abstract concrete peculiar
Judgment:	good (adequate) ←→ poor	good adequate poor
Estimated intelligence:	above average / average / borderline / retarded	above average / average / borderline / retarded
9. THOUGHT CONTENT		
Delusions:	grandiose / (persecutory) / somatic	grandiose / persecutory / somatic
Hallucinations:	yes (no)	yes no
Illusions & ideas reference	yes (no)	yes no
Obsessions & compulsions	yes (no)	yes no
Suicidal ideation:	(yes) no	yes no
Tombstone inscription:	REST IN PEACE	
Homicidal:	yes (no)	yes no
Motivation for treatment:	fair poor / (high)	fair poor / high
Insight:	fair (poor) / high	fair poor / high
T-shirt motto:		
What will you be doing two years from now?		
10. SENSORIUM		
Oriented for:	(time) / (place) / (person)	time / place / person
Memory impaired?	(yes) SOME no	yes no
General knowledge:	good (adequate) poor	good adequate poor

Form FPP-15-4/4-rev2/94 ©1994 GMS. Limited permission to photocopy only. For orders call (510) 865-5282, fax (510) 865-4295.

Mental Status Examination Glossary
For a definition of clinical terms

This abridged glossary has been prepared to save you time searching for definitions to some of the more arcane words used in the Mental Status Examination. I have tried to provide simpler, accurate definitions of what is found in clinical dictionaries.

Mental Status Examination Glossary
(page 1 of 2)

CONFABULATING

Falsification of memory occurring in clear consciousness in association with an organically determined amnesia. In psychiatry, **the act of replacing memory loss with fantasy or reality that is not true for the occasion.** The term also implies lack of insight, in the sense that the individual fully believes his answers. Confabulation is found in organic brain diseases in which intellectual impairment is a prominent feature.

DELUSION

A false belief that is firmly maintained even though it is contradicted by social reality. While it is true that some superstitions and religious beliefs are held despite the lack of confirmatory evidence, such culturally engendered concepts are not considered delusions. What is characteristic of the delusion is that it is not shared by others; rather, it is an idiosyncratic and individual misconception or misinterpretation. Further, it is a thinking disorder of enough import to interfere with the individual's functioning, since the area of delusion does not share a consensually validated reality with other people.

ECHOLALIA

Pathological imitation or repetition of another's speech, sometimes found in organic and schizophrenic disorders.

ECHOPRAXIA

Pathological repetition and imitation of another person's movements, sometimes found in organic and schizophrenic disorders.

FLIGHT OF IDEAS

A pathological speech pattern wherein the individual shifts rapidly from topic to topic.

HALLUCINATION

A false sense of perception, for example of an external object that does not actually exist.

IDEA OF REFERENCE

A false belief that other people's remarks, facial expressions, or gestures are always relating to oneself.

Form FPP-16-1/2-rev2/94 ©1994 GMS. Limited permission to photocopy only. For orders call (510) 865-5282, fax (510) 865-4295.

Mental Status Examination Glossary
(page 2 of 2)

ILLUSION	**A false perception,** such as that of a knife "bending" in water.
LABILITY	**The display of a wide range of emotions,** generally uncontrolled.
NEOLALIA	**The making up of words, or the fusion of words.**
NEOLOGISM	**Made-up words,** which are often condensations of other words, and may have a special meaning for the individual.
PERSEVERATION	**1. An individual's inability to shift from one task to another; 2. When an individual appears to respond to a question previously asked, but cannot respond to new or additional questions;** found in organic or schizophrenic disorders.
STEREOTYPY	**The repetition of any motion or action,** such as continuously rubbing a part of the body.
VERBIGERATION	Sometimes called cataphasia. **The continuous repetition of words or sentences.**

Client Billing Record I and II
For use in tracking what the patient owes

Many forms use the word *patient*, not *client*, because insurance companies are used to seeing the term *patient* in their records. Since billing records will most often be kept for insurance and IRS purposes, they feel it is simpler if the word *patient* is retained. In the forms included here the word client has been used uniformly throughout.

Two formats of billing records are included here, one to be used in a 5x8 binder, the other to be used in a standard 8½x11 binder. These binder sizes can be found at any stationery store.

The top of each billing record is filled out with the patient's name, address, coded ID number, referral source, date of referral, the billing diagnosis coded to DSM-III-R, and the year of billing. By using a three-column system, you will be able to see where you stand in relation to making payments and accounts receivable.

Some clinicians place billing records inside the patient's folder. Others prefer to keep them in separate binders so that financial records are separate from clinical notations. This latter method accomplishes two purposes. First, you don't have to weed through numerous records to get to billing information. Second, for purposes of confidentiality you can separate clinical notations from economic records relating to the same patient.

In addition to billing records, for an overall view of your practice you can keep a book that lists your total income for the day, adding each succeeding day of practice. Thus, at any given day of the year you can see your total income to date and any increase or decrease in your cash flow.

BILLING RECORD

Page: *1*

Client's Name: *MICHELLE SILVER*	Referred by:
Spouse's Name: *N/A*	Date of Referral:
Address: *1234 LANDS END AVE, SANTA MONICA, CA 90404*	Billing Diagnosis: *307.42 / 296.33*
Client's ID No. *92-SIL-01*	Year: *1992*

Date of Service	Client(s)	Amt. Billed	Amt. Paid	Balance Due
9 26	*MICHELLE*	*9 0 —*	*9 0 —*	*0 —*
9 30	*"*	*9 0 —*		*9 0 —*
10 2	*"*	*9 0 —*		*1 8 0 —*
10 9	*"*	*9 0 —*		*2 7 0 —*
10 16	*"*	*9 0 —*	*2 7 0 —*	*9 0 —*
10 23	*MICHELLE WITH MOTHER*	*9 0 —*		*1 8 0 —*
10 30	*MICHELLE*	*9 0 —*		*2 7 0 —*
11 6	*"*	*9 0 —*	*2 7 0 —*	*9 0 —*
11 13	*"*	*9 0 —*		*1 8 0 —*
11 20	*"*	*9 0 —*		*2 7 0 —*

BILLING RECORD

Page: 1

Client's Name: *MICHELLE SILVER*
Referred by:

Spouse's Name: *N/A*
Date of Referral:

Address: *1234 LANDS END AVE, SANTA MONICA, CA 90404*
Billing Diagnosis: *307.42/296.33*

Client's ID No. *92-SIL-01*
Year: *1992*

Date of Service	Client(s)	Amt. Billed	Amt. Paid	Balance Due
9 26	MICHELLE	90 —	90 —	0 —
9 30	"	90 —		90 —
10 2	"	90 —		180 —
10 9	"	90 —		270 —
10 16	"	90 —	270 —	90 —
10 23	MICHELLE WITH MOTHER	90 —		180 —
10 30	MICHELLE	90 —		270 —
11 6	"	90 —	270 —	90 —
11 13	"	90 —		180 —
11 20	"	90 —		270 —

Form FPP-18-1/1-rev2/94 ©1994 GMS. Limited permission to photocopy only. For orders call (510) 865-5282, fax (510) 865-4295.

BILLING RECORD

Page: 2

Client's Name: *MICHELLE SILVER*
Referred by:

Spouse's Name: *N/A*
Date of Referral:

Address: *1234 LANDS END AVE, SANTA MONICA, CA 90404*
Billing Diagnosis: *307.42/296.33*

Client's ID No.
Year: *1992-1993*

Date of Service	Client(s)	Amt. Billed	Amt. Paid	Balance Due
11 27	MICHELLE	90 —	270 —	90 —
12 4	"	90 —		180 —
12 11	"	90 —		270 —
12 18	"	90 —		360 —
1 5			360 —	0 —

Form FPP-18-1/1-rev2/94 ©1994 GMS. Limited permission to photocopy only. For orders call (510) 865-5282, fax (510) 865-4295.

Billing Statements I and II and the Superbill
For billing the patient or insurance carrier

Here you will see two separate billing statements and a sample of a personalized Superbill, which is also available on NCR (no carbon required) paper in triplicate. It is best to send your billing statements or a superbill on a one- to three-month cycle during the course of therapy.

Billing Statement I or II can be sent directly to the patient, attached to the provider's insurance form, or sent independently to an insurance provider. Insurance companies tend to frown on clinicians who submit a separate bill for each session.

The cost of processing forms for insurance companies, as well as the time it takes to fill out the simplest of superbills, can impact the cost effectiveness of your practice and leave you far less time to do the work you are trained to do. Insurance company hotlines have provided estimates of processing costs that range from $3.00 to $7.50 per billing statement. In an era of cost containment, this should be considered in your billing practices.

Billing Statement I contains Current Procedural Terminology (CPT) codes; Billing Statement II does not. CPT codes are updated yearly. A complete CPT code book can be obtained from the American Medical Association. These forms have been designed with and without codes, depending on whether they will be used by a medical or nonmedical clinician.

Depending on the size of your practice, there may not be a great deal of difference in using Billing Statements I or II and the Superbill. Billing Statements I and II require more written information, as you must enter both diagnostic and procedural codes. The need to maintain a copy of this form requires photocopying.

The Superbill will save you time because it includes both CPT codes and diagnostic coding and is in NCR triplicate format. A cost-effectiveness study of both formats after one year would let you know which is more effective for your practice. In the beginning, try both ways. It is worth the initial investment and will help you in developing a record-keeping and billing style that suits your specific needs.

Date: *11-21-92*	**STATEMENT**

To: *NATIONAL INSURANCE CO. 2780 CENTRAL BLVD., LOS ANGELES, CA 90066*

Name of Insured: *MICHELLE SILVER*

Address: *1234 LANDS END AVE.*

City: *SANTA MONICA*   State: *CA*   Zip: *90404*

Name of Client: *MICHELLE SILVER*   Relationship to Insured: *SELF*

Referring Physician: Date:

The following professional services were provided to the above-named client as itemized, and on the dates listed below, for the diagnosis of: *307.42 / 296.33*

DATE	SERVICE RENDERED		CHARGE
	Procedure Code	Description	
9.26.92	*90844*	*INDIVIDUAL 50 MINUTES*	*90 —*
9.30.92	*"*	*" "*	*90 —*
10.2.92	*"*	*" "*	*90 —*
10.9.92	*"*	*" "*	*90 —*
10.16.92	*"*	*" "*	*90 —*
10.23.92	*90847*	*CONJOINT "*	*90 —*
10.30.92	*90844*	*INDIVIDUAL "*	*90 —*
11.6.92	*"*	*" "*	*90 —*
11.13.92	*"*	*" "*	*90 —*
11.20.92	*"*	*" "*	*90 —*

Clinician's Signature: *George R. Jones, Ph.D.*	**TOTAL:**
Soc. Sec. No./Fed. ID No. *999-99-9999*	*900.00*
State License Number: *K.Y. 5011*	

Form FPP-19-1/1-rev2/94 ©1994 GMS. Limited permission to photocopy only. For orders call (510) 865-5282, fax (510) 865-4295.

Date: 11-21-92	STATEMENT		

		DIAGNOSIS	
Name of Insured: MICHELLE SILVER			
Address: 1234 LANDS END AVE.	Axis I 307.42/296.33		
	Axis II 799.90		
SANTA MONICA, CA 90404	Axis III SEE MED. REPORT		
Name of Client: MICHELLE SILVER	Axis IV 4		
	Axis V(a) 40		
Relationship to Insured: SELF	Axis V(b) 50-60		

Date	Service Rendered		Total Fee	Balance
	* Procedure	Description		
9-26-92	90844	INDIVIDUAL 50 MINUTES	90 -	90 -
9-30-92	"	" "	90 -	180 -
10-2-92	"	" "	90 -	270 -
10-9-92	"	" "	90 -	360 -
10-16-92	"	" "	90 -	450 -
10-23-92	90847	CONJOINT "	90 -	540 -
10-30-92	90844	INDIVIDUAL "	90 -	630 -
11-6-92	"	" "	90 -	720 -
11-13-92	"	" "	90 -	810 -
11-20-92	"	" "	90 -	900 -
			Balance Now Due	900 -

* No.	Procedure	CPT
1	Individual 50 minutes	90844
2	Individual 25 minutes	90843
3	Family/Conjoint	90847
4	Multiple-Family	90849
5	Group	90853
6	Report Preparation	90889
7	Diagnostic Interview	90801
8	Testing, with Report	90830
9	Telephone Consultation	98920

Clinician's Signature: George R. Jones, Ph.D.

SSN or Federal ID Number. 999-99-9999

State License No. X.Y.5011

Form FPP-20-1/1-rev2/94 ©1994 GMS. Limited permission to photocopy only. For orders call (510) 865-5282, fax (510) 865-4295.

Superbill

Superbills have been used by medical specialists since about 1985, and they are now creeping into our field. The advantages of using a superbill over filling out a statement or an insurance form are numerous. Superbills can be specialized for your practice. They are easily and quickly filled out by hand, and the Superbill given here can be used for 1 to 10 sessions. This Superbill differs from the many available that are designed for only one session.

This Superbill has simplified DSM-III-R diagnostic codes and CPT codes. It is available in triplicate: the original for the insurance company, and a copy each for you and your client, respectively.

If this particular Superbill fits your needs, you may order packs of it using the order form in the back of this book.

SUPERBILL

DSM-III-R DIAGNOSIS

DEVELOPMENTAL DISORDERS DSM-III-R:	DISSOCIATIVE DISORDERS DSM-III-R:
ORGANIC MENTAL DISORDERS DSM-III-R:	SEXUAL DISORDERS DSM-III-R:
SUBSTANCE USE DISORDER DSM-III-R:	SLEEP DISORDERS DSM-III-R:
SCHIZOPHRENIA DSM-III-R:	FACTITIOUS DISORDERS DSM-III-R:
DELUSIONAL DISORDER DSM-III-R:	IMPULSE CONTROL DISORDERS DSM-III-R:
PSYCHOTIC DISORDERS DSM-III-R:	ADJUSTMENT DISORDERS DSM-III-R:
MOOD DISORDERS DSM-III-R:	PSY FACTORS AFFECTING PHYS COND DSM-III-R:
ANXIETY DISORDERS DSM-III-R:	PERSONALITY DISORDERS DSM-III-R:
SOMATOFORM DISORDERS DSM-III-R:	V CODES DSM-III-R:

	DATE OF SERVICE	CPT CODE	CHARGES
1.	9-26-92	90844	90 -
2.	9-30-92	''	90 -
3.	10-2-92	''	90 -
4.	10-9-92	''	90 -
5.	10-16-92	''	90 -
6.	10-23-92	90847	90 -
7.	10-30-92	90844	90 -
8.	11-6-92	''	90 -
9.	11-13-92	''	90 -
10.	11-20-92	''	90 -
		TOTAL	900.00

POLICY HOLDER	INSURANCE CARRIER	POLICY NUMBER
MICHELLE SILVER	National Insurance Co.	MED3218234

POLICY HOLDER'S SSN	ADDRESS	CITY STATE ZIP
222-22-2222	1234 LANDS END AVE	SANTA MONICA CA 90404

CLIENT'S NAME Circle M (F)	RELATIONSHIP TO POLICY HOLDER	CLIENT'S BIRTHDATE
MICHELLE SILVER	SELF	9-21-58

REFERRED BY	DATE SYMPTOM FIRST OCCURRED	LOCATION SERVICES RENDERED
	8-26-92	OFFICE ✓ OTHER

AUTHORIZATION TO PROVIDE INFORMATION TO INSURANCE CARRIER:
I HEREBY AUTHORIZE THE RELEASE OF ANY INFORMATION ACQUIRED IN THE COURSE OF MY EXAMINATION AND TREATMENT.
SIGNATURE Michelle Silver DATE 11-21-92

AUTHORIZATION TO ASSIGN BENEFITS TO PROVIDER:
I CERTIFY THAT THE SERVICES LISTED HAVE BEEN RECEIVED AND I AUTHORIZE PAYMENT TO BE MADE DIRECTLY TO SAID CLINICIAN.
SIGNATURE Michelle Silver DATE 11-21-92

PROCEDURE CODES	
90844 45–50 MINUTES	
HOSPITAL CARE	90847 FAMILY PSYCHOTHERAPY
90200 BRIEF HIST AND EXAM	90849 MULT FAM GRP PSYCHOTHERAPY
90215 INTERMEDIATE HIST AND EXAM	90853 GROUP PSYCHOTHERAPY
90220 COMPREHENSIVE HIST AND EXAM	90870 ECT: SINGLE SEIZURE
90240 EACH DAY, BRIEF SERVICES	90871 MULT SEIZURES PER DAY
90250 LIMITED SERVICES	90880 HYPNOTHERAPY
90260 INTERMEDIATE SERVICES	90882 ENVIRONMENTAL INTERVENTION
90270 EXTENDED SERVICES	90887 INTERPRET OF EXAM RESULTS
90280 COMPREHENSIVE SERVICES	90889 UNLISTED PROCEDURE
90292 HOSPITAL DISCHARGE	*BIOFEEDBACK*
THERAPEUTIC INJECTIONS	90900 BIOFEEDBACK TRAINING
90782 INJECTION OF MEDICATION	90904 REG OF BLOOD PRESSURE
SPECIFY:	90906 REG OF SKIN TEMP
90784 INTRAVENOUS	90908 BY EEG APPLICATION
INTERVIEW PROCEDURES	**MEDICAL PROCEDURE CODES**
90801 DIAGNOSTIC INTERVIEW EXAM	*OFFICE VISITS*
90825 EVALUATION RECS OR REPORTS	90020 INIT COMPREHENSIVE EVAL
90830 PSYCHOLOGICAL TESTING	90060 INTERMEDIATE VISIT
90831 TELEPHONE CONSULTATION	90070 EXTENDED VISIT
90835 NARCOSYNTHESIS	*HOSPITAL CONSULTATIONS*
THERAPEUTIC PROCEDURES	90620 INITIAL, COMPREHENSIVE
90841 INDIV. PSYCHOTHERAPY; UNSPEC	90630 INITIAL, COMPLEX
90843 20–30 MINUTES	90643 FOLLOW-UP

11-21-92
TODAY'S DATE

George R. Jones
PROVIDER'S SIGNATURE

X.Y.5011   PSYCHOLOGIST
TYPE OF LICENSE, STATE LICENSE NUMBER

999-99-9999
PROVIDER'S FEDERAL TAX ID OR SSN

Insurance Provider's Form
For billing the insurance provider

The Blue Shield of California health insurance claim form that is reproduced here is typical of most forms provided by insurance companies for reimbursement of services. Ask patients to fill out the subscriber information section of the insurance form. Then attach it to a billing statement or superbill, and submit it to the insurance company for direct reimbursement. If you wish to have reimbursement made directly to you, be sure that the equivalent of item 13 is signed by the patient or the patient's authorized representative. The sections of a typical insurance form are described below.

This form should be typed whenever possible. However, forms clearly filled out in blue or black ink are accepted by insurance companies.

1. **Patient's name** (first name, middle initial, last name).

2. **Patient's date of birth.**

3. **Subscriber's name.** The subscriber and the patient may not be the same person. For example, you may see a woman whose husband is the subscriber; she is covered by his policy.

4. **Patient's address** (street, city, state, zip code).

5. **Patient's sex.** Although I have always believed that this should be noted as the patient's gender, we live in an age when transsexuals may wish to be considered a gender opposite from their birth gender. Have your client check with the insurance company if these gender issues occur so that you can respond based on the insurance company's protocol.

6. **Subscriber's number.** Remember this is the *subscriber's* number, not the patient's number. Typically, this number will be a social security number.

7. **Patient's relationship to subscriber.** Note that there are political and social movements to allow homosexuals couples the right to carry dependent partners on the insurance policy of the policy holder, in the same way a heterosexual spouse can be carried. Calling your client's insurance company and speaking with the physicians' claims representative will help you to determine whether a

INSURANCE PROVIDER'S FORM

Patient (Subscriber) Information		
1. Patient's Name (First, Middle Initial, Last) *MICHELLE SILVER*	2. Patient's D.O.B. *9-21-58*	3. Subscriber Name (First, Middle Initial, Last) *MICHELLE SILVER*
4. Patient's Address (Street, city, state, zip) *1234 LANDS END AVE.* *SANTA MONICA, CA 90404*	5. Patient's Sex: Male (Female)	6. Subscriber No. *99999*
	7. Patient's relationship to subscriber: (Self) Spouse Child Other	8. Subscriber's Group (Or Group No.) *MED 3218234*
9. If other health insurance coverage: enter Name and ID No. of policyholder; Employer's name; and Insuring Company's name and address	10. Was condition related to: A. Patient's Employment (Yes) No B. Auto Accident (Yes) No	11. Subscriber's Address (Street, city, state, zip) *1234 LANDS END AVE.* *SANTA MONICA, CA 90404*
12. I Authorize the Release of any Medical Information Necessary to Process this Claim. *Michelle Silver* Signed (insured or authorized person)	13. I Authorize Payment of Medical Benefits to Undersigned or Supplier for Services Described Below. *Michelle Silver* Signed (insured or authorized person)	

Physician or Supplier Information								
14. Date of *8-26-92*	Illness (first symptom) or Injury (accident) or Pregnancy	15. Date you first consulted your physician *9-26-92*	16. Has patient ever had same or similar symptoms? Yes (No)				
17. Date able to return to work *10-1-92*	18. Dates of total disability From Through	Dates of partial disability From Through						
19. Name and address of referring physician or other source	20. For hospital services, please give dates Admitted Discharged						
21. Name and address of facility where services rendered (if other than home or office)	22. Was lab work performed outside your office? Yes (No) Charges?						

23. Diagnosis or nature of illness or injury. (Relate diagnosis to procedure below by reference to numbers 1, 2, 3, etc., or DX code)
1. *307.42* } AXIS I
2. *296.33*
3. *799.90 – AXIS II*
4.

24. Service Date	Place	Procedure #	Fully describe services or supplies given each date	Code	Charges	Balance
9-26-92	3	90844	INDIVIDUAL PSYCHOTHERAPY	1,2	90 –	90 –
9-30-92	3	90844	" "	1,2	90 –	180 –
10-2-92	3	90844	" "	1,2	90 –	270 –
10-9-92	3	90844	" "	1,2	90 –	360 –
10-16-92	3	90844	" "	1,2	90 –	450 –
10-23-92	3	90844	" "	1,2	90 –	540 –
10-30-92	3	90844	" "	1,2	90 –	630 –
11-6-92	3	90844	" "	1,2	90 –	720 –

25. Signature of physician or supplier Signed *George R. Jones* *11-7-92* Dated	26. Accept Assignment Yes No	27. Total Assign. *720 –*	28. Amt. Paid *0 –*	29. Balance Due *720 –*
	30. Social Security No. *999-99-9999*	31. Physician's or supplier's name, address, provider number, and telephone number *GEORGE R. JONES*			
32. Patient's Account No. *92-SIL-01*	33. Your Employer ID No. *99-5555*			

Codes: 1(IH)-Inpatient Hospital, 2(OH)-Outpatient Hospital, 3(O)- Doctor's Office, 4(H)-Patient's Home, 5-Day Care Facility, 6-Night Care Facility	7(ICF)-Intermediate Care Facility, 8(SNF)-Skilled Nursing Facility, 9-Ambulance, O(OL)-Other Locations, A-Indep. Laboratory, B-Other	*929 W. MAIN BLVD. STE. 101* *LOS ANGELES, CA 90000* *X.Y.5011 (213) 555-7927*

Form FPP-22-1/1-rev2/94 ©1994 GMS. Do not reproduce. For orders call (510) 865-5282, fax (510) 865-4295.

homosexual partner is entitled to the benefits of the significant other. However, I suggest you obtain a signed release of information from your client or have the client speak to the company when this issue arises.

8. **Subscriber's group number** (or group name). The group number typically applies to the type of coverage the plan offers. Many insurance companies require prior authorization before paying for provision of services. Contact the company's claims representative for information.

9. **If other health insurance coverage** (Enter name and I.D. number of policyholder, and insuring company's name and address). Insurance companies are now coordinating the payment of services so that the provider and the patient cannot receive more money than the total bill. I disagree with this procedure, since policies are paid for as if there is only one provider. I believe the insurance industry should reimburse the full amount or offer a premium reduction to people who are covered under two policies. Until they do, it seems equitable that insurance companies should pay the full amount for the services that are being paid for by the patient or the patient's employer. Overages could then be given directly to the patient to cover other services that may not be covered under the policy. Or, companies could use the overages to reduce insurance premiums or add better coverage to their existing policies.

10. **Was condition related to: A. Patient's employment, B. Accident**. This section is extremely important. Many policies will not issue benefits if, in the insurer's opinion, the injury reported could relate to a worker's compensation claim, a disability claim, or be paid for by someone else's insurance company, such as an auto accident in which the other person is at fault.

11. **Subscriber's address** (street, city, state, zip code). This is the subscriber's—not necessarily the client's—address.

12. **I authorize the release of any medical information necessary to process this claim** (patient's or authorized person's signature). I believe that, ethically, you should explain to patients that an insurance company paying for the services of psychotherapy has a right to all clinical notations, test results, and any other clinical information relating to the case. Explain this up front so they can decide whether or not they wish to use their insurance. Some clinicians advise their patients not to submit to their insurance company

claims for tests such as the MMPI so that particular part of the record will not be required to be reported. However, all records are subject to subpoena.

13. **I authorize payment of medical benefits to undersigned physician or supplier for services described below.** This signature is optional.

14. **Date of illness (first symptoms) or injury (accident) or pregnancy (LMP).** This is the date the symptoms first occurred. If you are seeing a patient who has had previous psychotherapy, the insurance company may categorize it as a preexisting condition and refuse to cover it. Check the date and diagnosis of any and all claims that the patient submitted prior to seeing you. Specifically check whether payments came from other insurance carriers. Most waivers for preexisting conditions last from two to five years.

15. **Date first consulted you for this condition.**

16. **Has patient ever had same or similar symptoms?** This question relates directly to the discussion in item 14.

17. **Date patient able to return to work.**

18. **Dates of total disability from . . . through . . . Dates of partial disability, from . . . through . . .** This designation can be made only by some practitioners. In California, disabilities are typically the province of clinical psychologists and psychiatrists. If you need to fill in these spaces and you are not a clinical psychologist or a psychiatrist, you will probably need one to designate dates for you.

19. **Name and address of referring physician or other source.**

20. **For services related to hospitalization give hospital dates: admitted, discharged.**

21. **Name and address of facility where services rendered** (if other than home or office). This is the location where you are providing the service. This space need not be filled in unless the location is other than your home or office.

22. **Was laboratory work performed outside your office?**

23. **Diagnosis or nature of illness or injury. Relate diagnosis to procedure in column D by reference to numbers 1, 2, 3, etc. or DX code.** Most forms are not designed to accommodate the multiaxial diagnosis as required in reporting using the DSM-III-R. I

recommend that you use Axis I diagnoses and Axis II diagnoses. Axis III diagnoses should be noted when a medical condition is, in your professional opinion, related to either an Axis I or II diagnosis.

24. **Date of service.**

Place of service.

Fully describe procedures, medical services or supplies furnished for each date given (explain unusual services or circumstances). Procedure code. This is typically filled in with the word *psychotherapy* and the procedure number. Procedure numbers come from the physicians' *Current Procedural Terminology* manual. This manual can be purchased from the American Medical Association, Department of Coding and Nomenclature, 515 North State Street, Chicago, IL 60610. The cost of a CPT manual and supplement varies from year to year. In general, you will probably spend no more than $25.

Diagnosis code. If your procedure differs based on the fact that you have two separate diagnoses on Axis I, remember to refer to item 24 so that the procedure is related to the diagnostic code. An example: On Axis I of the DSM-III-R diagnosis, you may have indicated dysthymia (300.40) and a marital problem (V61.10). In the space of 24C, you may refer to individual psychotherapy with its CPT number of 908.44; and in relation to the marital V-code, you may wish to refer to the CPT code of 908.47, which is conjoint marital psychotherapy.

Charges. This is the charge per session and should be filled in as indicated on the sample form.

25. **Signature of physician or supplier:** *I certify under penalty that the foregoing is true and correct.* This section is self-explanatory, except when you are be signing for your intern. Under those circumstances, the intern should sign first with his or her degree and intern number. Then write "Supervised by" and sign your name, with your degree and license number. An example:

> Jerome Bower, M.A., I.N. J123450
> Supervised by:
> Michael I. Gold, Ph.D., XY1234

26. **Accept assignment.** This is an agreement regarding whether or not you will accept what the insurance company pays in full. As you can see, the form includes the phrase "government claims only."

Pending legislation may soon require clinicians dealing with government payments for services to have special provider numbers or preapproval of services before payment will be made.

27. **Total charge**.

28. **Amount paid**.

29. **Balance due**.

30. **Social security number**. Your social security number or taxpayer's identification number should be put on all forms even when an intern is providing the direct services.

31. **Physician's or supplier's name, address, zip code, telephone number, and I.D. number** (Provider number). This should be typed as follows:

    ACB 00 M ZZZ12345M AC *(provider number)*
    Michael I. Gold, Ph.D., MFCC (XY1234)
    1234 Main Boulevard, Suite 15
    Los Angeles, CA 90000

Often, you will be an authorized provider, which means that your name will be printed in a directory of clinicians who are willing to accept the particular insurance company's payment in full for services rendered. Insurance companies will typically provide you with their forms, preprinted with your provider information.

Provider or I.D. numbers, depending on the agency, refer to your social security number or federal tax I.D. number. Sometimes, however, insuring companies issue special provider numbers. When you are requested to give your provider or I.D. number, check with the company or agency about which is the appropriate number to use.

32. **Patient's account number**. As discussed in the section on the Confidential Patient Information form, one system of giving each patient an account number is as follows: the year of service, the first three letters of the patient's last name, and 01. For example, Jerome Bower's account number would be: 92-BOW-01.

If another patient whose last name is Bower were to enter the practice in the same year, the designation of the third section of the coding system would be increased by one: 92-BOW-02.

33. **Employer I.D. number**. For those of you working with agencies, obtain this number from the accounting department.

4

When There Are Special Circumstances
Forms to Be Used in Special Circumstances

The forms on the following pages are used on an intermittent basis, monthly or yearly, depending on your patients.

For example, suppose that while you are seeing a patient, the patient is injured in an accident, then sues or is being sued. This will often require your direct participation in writing reports, appearing as an expert witness, being deposed about the psychological condition of the patient, or being required to provide a copy of your billing records.

Remember, the clients you are seeing now—whatever their issues—may involve you in a legal situation later. That is why the forms in Chapter 4 are extremely important. Be sure to check with your state agency or association about forms (such as a child abuse reporting form) that you must have at your disposal.

Authorization to Obtain Confidential Information
For the privilege of obtaining confidential data

This form is to be used *at all times* before speaking with anyone with regard to a client. Confidentiality, as well as privilege, remains with the client whenever you are in doubt. Check with your state board or state professional association for any exceptions to this rule. In the state of California, for example, unless special circumstances exist, if you are called regarding any client in your caseload, you must state that you can neither confirm nor deny the existence of this person as your client.

AUTHORIZATION TO OBTAIN CONFIDENTIAL INFORMATION

I, ___Michelle Silver___ , hereby authorize and request that
(Client's Name)

___Cynthia Roberts, Ph.D - Paige Psychological Services___
(Name of Information Source)

___8765 West Street, Los Angeles, CA 91234___
(Address and Phone Number)

may release all confidential medical, psychological, psychiatric, educational, and/or other appropriate information acquired in the course of my evaluations and treatments (or those of my minor children) to

___George Jones, Ph.D.___
(Clinician's Name)

I understand that I may revoke this consent at any time by informing the above parties in writing.

In consideration of this consent, I hereby release the above parties from any legal liability for the release of this information.

Signature ___Michelle Silver___ Date ___April 21, 1992___
(Client)

and/or

Signature _____ Date _____
(Parent or Guardian)

Form FPP-23-1/1-rev2/94 ©1994 GMS. Limited permission to photocopy only. For orders call (510) 865-5282, fax (510) 865-4295.

Consent for Release of Confidential Information
For authority to release confidential data

This convenient form has been designed as a fill-in form for your practice. It is straightforward and simple to use.

This form can also be used in couples and family counseling. Ask all parties involved in conjoint and family sessions to sign this release. This will make clear to them that you cannot hold confidentiality or privilege due to the possibility of triangulation, which can occur when doing therapy with more than one client.

In the history of my practice, I have been triangulated more than once by a simple two-minute phone call. This occurs when one of the clients calls to "secretly share some personal information." It has the potential of being perceived by other clients as my withholding and, therefore, betraying their trust.

I cannot emphasize strongly enough the need for this form to be signed by clients in conjoint family therapy.

CONSENT FOR RELEASE OF CONFIDENTIAL INFORMATION

I, _____Michelle Silver_____ hereby authorize and request that
   (Client's Name)

_____George Jones, Ph.D._____
   (Clinician's Name)

may release all confidential professional information pertaining to me (or my minor children) to

_____National Insurance Co._____

_____2780 Central Blvd._____

_____Los Angeles, CA 9066_____

I understand that I may revoke this consent at any time by informing the above parties

in writing.

In consideration of this consent, I hereby release the above parties from any legal

liability for the release of this information.

Signature _____Michelle Silver_____ Date _____April 21, 1992_____
   (Client)

and/or

Signature _____ Date _____
   (Parent or Guardian)

Clinical Consultations
For information gathered during a session

This form can be kept separate from the clinical notations in each client's folder. This form enables you to differentiate between information gathered from the client during a session and from tests administered, and information you receive from other clinicians and institutions.

CLINICAL CONSULTATIONS

CLIENT'S NAME: MICHELLE	CLIENT'S ID NO. 92-SIL-01	DATE: 1992

Date: 5-5-92	Consultant's Name: ROBERT YOUNG, MD	Profession: PYCHIATRIST
	Address: 2201 CENTER BLVD., LOS ANGELES, CA, 90000	
	Telephone: (213) 444-3333	
	Client's Release of Confidentiality signed: YES	Date: 5-5-92

PURPOSE OF CONSULT
☐ MEDICAL
☒ PSYCHIATRIC
☐ LEGAL
☐ TESTING
☐ SCHOOL
☐ OTHER

COMMENTS:

INFORM ME OF DIAGNOSIS AND MEDICATION.

PLUS RESULTS FROM REPORT.

Date: 10-22-93	Consultant's Name: CYNTHIA ROBERTS, Ph.D	Profession: PSYCHOLOGIST
	Address: 8765 WEST. ST., LOS ANGELES, CA 91234	
	Telephone: (213) 555-1963	
	Client's Release of Confidentiality signed: YES	Date: 10-22-93

PURPOSE OF CONSULT
☐ MEDICAL
☐ PSYCHIATRIC
☐ LEGAL
☒ TESTING
☐ SCHOOL
☐ OTHER

COMMENTS:

DISCUSSED TESTING RESULTS PREVIOUS TO

MENTAL HEALTH TREATMENT REPORT.

Date: 8-30-93	Consultant's Name: DAVID STEIN	Profession: ATTORNEY
	Address: 4625 PARK AVE.	
	Telephone: (213) 555-9988	
	Client's Release of Confidentiality signed: YES	Date: 8-30-93

PURPOSE OF CONSULT
☐ MEDICAL
☐ PSYCHIATRIC
☐ LEGAL
☐ TESTING
☐ SCHOOL
☐ OTHER

COMMENTS:

DISCUSSED WHAT EMPHASIS WAS NECESSARY

IN SUMMATION SECTION OF M.H.T.R.

Life-Threatening Behavior Scale
For evaluation of life-threatening behavior

Based on the research available, as well as my own clinical impressions, I have found that the opinion of the clinician is many times more valuable than the self-reporting of the client when evaluating suicidal potential. I have further found, when working with clients, that by introducing the concept of "life-threatening behavior" rather than suicidality, the inquiry becomes less charged, which allows for clearer information to be reported.

When interviewing clients regarding suicidality, I frequently say, "I am concerned about your committing suicide or taking your own life." When the return response is some form of denial that is dissonant with my clinical observations, I introduce the concept of "life-threatening behavior."

I use the example of smoking a cigarette. Smoking a cigarette may be life threatening eventually, so on a scale of 1 to 10 it would be rated as a 1. Drunk driving on a freeway, however, could be an 8 or 9.

What is often more helpful to the clinician than the actual average rating for each category is to consider the number of items entered in each category. For example, a score of 4–6 theoretically represents a medium degree of lethality. However, if the client only responds to one item in a category and ranks it 4–6, theoretically the client's life-threatening behavior ranks low.

What I find more significant are cases in which over 20 different items average a rating of 5. The mere fact that the client responds to many items that can affect suicidality is clinically more significant than the rating of any individual item. Certain items with a rating of 7–9 are also extremely significant. The rating scale proves most useful not only by giving an average rating but by clinically analyzing a specific rating in a specific time. Ultimately, this scale should be used with the most useful tool a clinician has—instinct.

Using the Life-Threatening Behavior Scale will help you confirm your clinical impressions and relate those impressions to other professionals or persons that you may have to contact in the event of a potential suicide. This scale was taken from the Atlanta Revision of the Los Angeles Suicide Potentiality Rating Scale.

LIFE-THREATENING BEHAVIOR SCALE (page 1 of 4)

CLIENT'S FIRST NAME: *MICHELLE*	CLIENT'S ID NO. *92-SIL-01*	AGE: *34*	SEX: *F*	DATE: *10-30-92*

RATER: *DR. JONES*	DEGREE OF LETHALITY: 1 2 3 ④ 5 6 7 8 9 LOW MEDIUM HIGH

This schedule attempts to rate suicide potentiality.

Listed below are categories with descriptive items that have been found to be useful in evaluating suicide potentiality. The numbers in parentheses after each item suggest the most common range of values or weights assigned to that item. Nine is the highest or MOST seriously suicidal, while 1 is the lowest or the LEAST seriously suicidal. The rating assigned will depend on the individual case. The rater should note that the range of numbers to be assigned will vary for each item.

The rating for each of the five categories is the average of the ratings assigned to the total number of items ranked within that category. (Seldom will one be able to rate every item.)

The overall suicide potentiality rating may be found by entering the rates assigned for each category, then totaling and dividing by the number of categories rated. This number, rounded to the nearest whole number, should be circled at the top of this page. It is this number (circled above) which represents the degree of lethality for the person being evaluated.

A. AGE AND SEX

	MALE	
1.	50 Plus (7–9)	
2.	35–49 (5–7)	
3.	15–34 (3–5)	
	FEMALE	
4.	All ages (1–3)	*1*
	RATING FOR CATEGORY A	*1*

LIFE-THREATENING BEHAVIOR SCALE (page 2 of 4)

CLIENT'S FIRST NAME: *MICHELLE*	CLIENT'S ID NO. *92-SIL-01*	DATE: *10-30-92*

B. SYMPTOMS

1.	Severe depression: sleep disorder, anorexia, weight loss, withdrawal, despondency, loss of interest, apathy. (7–9)	*9*
2.	Feelings of hopelessness, helplessness, exhaustion. (7–9)	*9*
3.	Disorganization, confusion, chaos, delusions, hallucinations, loss of contact, disorientation. (5–8)	*N/R* *
4.	Alcoholism, drug addiction, homosexuality, compulsive gambling. (4–8)	*N/R*
5.	Agitation, tension, anxiety. (4–6)	*5*
6.	Guilt, shame, embarrassment. (4–6)	*6*
7.	Feelings of rage, hostility, anger, revenge, jealousy. (4–6)	*6*
8.	Poor impulse control, poor judgment. (4–6)	*4*
9.	Chronic debilitating illness. (5–7)	*5*
10.	Repeated unsuccessful experiences with doctors or therapists. (4–6)	*N/R*
11.	Psychosomatic illness (asthma, ulcers, etc.) or hypochondria (chronic minor illness complaints). (1–4)	*4*
	SUM OF CATEGORY B	*48*

THE SUM OF CATEGORY B __*48*__ DIVIDED BY THE NUMBER OF ITEMS RATED __*8*__
EQUALS THE AVERAGE RATING FOR CATEGORY B __*6*__ .

* *NOT RATED*

LIFE-THREATENING BEHAVIOR SCALE   (page 3 of 4)

CLIENT'S FIRST NAME: *Michelle*	CLIENT'S ID NO. *92-SIL-01*	DATE: *10-30-92*

C. STRESS AND ITS OCCURRENCE (Acute vs Chronic)

1.	Loss of loved person by death, divorce, or separation (including possible long-term hospitalization, etc). (5–9)	N/R
2.	Loss of job, money, prestige, status. (4–8)	8
3.	Sickness, serious illness, surgery, accident, loss of limb. (3–7)	6
4.	Threat of prosecution, criminal involvement, exposure. (4–6)	N/R
5.	Change(s) in life, environment, setting. (4–6)	5
6.	Sharp, noticeable, and sudden onset of specific stress symptoms. (1–9)	8
7.	Recurrent outbreak of similar symptoms or stress. (4–9)	6
8.	Recent increase in long-standing traits, symptoms, or stress. (1–9)	6
	SUM OF CATEGORY D	39

THE SUM OF CATEGORY C __39__ DIVIDED BY THE NUMBER OF ITEMS RATED __6__
EQUALS THE AVERAGE RATING FOR CATEGORY C __6__ .

D. PRIOR SUICIDAL BEHAVIOR AND CURRENT PLAN

1.	Rate lethality of previous attempts. (1–9)	N/R
2.	History of repeated threats and depression. (3–5)	3
3.	Specificity of current plan and lethality of proposed method: aspirin, pills, poison, knife, drowning, hanging, jumping, gun. (1–9)	N/R
4.	Availability of means for proposed method and specificity in time planned. (1–9)	N/R
	SUM OF CATEGORY D	3

THE SUM OF CATEGORY D __3__ DIVIDED BY THE NUMBER OF ITEMS RATED __1__
EQUALS THE AVERAGE RATING FOR CATEGORY D __3__ .

LIFE THREATENING BEHAVIOR SCALE (page 4 of 4)

CLIENT'S FIRST NAME: *MICHELLE*	CLIENT'S ID NO. 92-SIL-01	DATE: 10-30-92

E. RESOURCES, COMMUNICATION ASPECTS, AND REACTION OF SIGNIFICANT OTHERS

1.	No sources of financial support (employment, agencies, family). (4–9)	6
2.	No personal emotional support: family or friends unavailable, unwilling to help. (4–7)	7
3.	Communication broken by others with rejection of patient's efforts to reestablish relationships. (5–7)	N/R
4.	Communications have internalized goal, e.g., declaration of guilt; feelings of worthlessness, blame, shame. (4–7)	6
5.	Communications have interpersonalized goal, e.g., to cause guilt in others, to force action in others. (2–4)	2

Reaction of Significant Others*

6.	Defensive, paranoid, rejecting, punishing attitude. (5–7)	NOT INTERVIEWED
7.	Denial of own or patient's need for help. (5–7)	N/I
8.	No feeling of concern about the patient; does not understand the patient. (4–6)	N/I
9.	Indecisive or alternating attitude—feelings of anger and rejection and of responsibility and desire to help. (2–5)	N/I
* Answers gained by direct contact with significant other(s) are often more reliable than those gained from the patient.	SUM OF CATEGORY E	21

THE SUM OF CATEGORY E ___21___ DIVIDED BY THE NUMBER OF ITEMS RATED ___4___
EQUALS THE AVERAGE RATING FOR CATEGORY E ___5___ .

CATEGORY	RATING
A. Age and Sex	1
B. Symptoms	6
C. Stress and Its Occurrence	6
D. Prior Suicidal Behavior and Current Plan	3
E. Resources, Communication Aspects, and Reaction of Significant Others	5
TOTAL:	21
DIVIDE by the number of categories rated	5
AVERAGE (round to the nearest whole number and circle at the top of the first page at degree of lethality)	4

Adapted from the Atlanta Revision of the Los Angeles Suicide Potentiality Rating Scale.

Suspected Child Abuse Report
For reporting child abuse as required by the state

The necessity of reporting certain information gathered in a clinical setting differs from state to state. In California and many other states, clinicians are required to report suspected child abuse. Included here is a sample form modeled on the one put out by the Child Abuse Hotline.

I check with the hotline worker to see if a particular incident should be reported, then fill out this form in the presence of the person informing me and with the aid of the hotline worker. Professionals working for child protective services are very cooperative in aiding with this procedure.

Check with your licensing board, state association, or the child protective services in the city where you are practicing to see if such forms are available. They will inform you about the availability and distribution of the forms. Typically, there is a time frame involved, beginning with reporting the incident over the phone to the time by which the form must be mailed.

SUSPECTED CHILD ABUSE REPORT

A. Case Identification (to be completed by the investigating CPA)

Victim Name *JENKINS, CHARLES*   Report No./Case Name_____ Date *1-17-94*

B. Reporting Party

Name/Title *GEORGE R. JONES , Ph. D., MFCC*

Address *929 W. MAIN BLVD., STE. 101, LOS ANGELES, CA 90000*

Phone *(213)555-7927* | Date of Report *1-17-94* | Signature of Reporting Party *George R. Jones*

C. Report Sent To

☐ Police Department   ☐ Sheriff's Office   ☐ County Welfare   ☐ County Probation

Agency *DEPT. OF CHILDREN'S SERVICES* | Address *12 CENTER ST., LOS ANGELES, CA 94808*

Official Contacted *WILLIAM BLAS, MSW* | Phone *(213) 555-2231* | Date/Time *1-7-94 6³⁰PM*

D. Involved Parties: Victim

Name (last, first, middle) *JENKINS, CHARLES* | Address *21 2nd ST. LOS ANGELES* | D.O.B. *8-26-87* | Sex *M* | Race *C*

Present Location of Child *ST. LUKES HOSPITAL, 3 WILSHIRE, LOS ANGELES* | Phone *(213) 555-7742*

D. Involved Parties: Siblings

Name *NONE*   D.O.B   Sex   Race   Name   D.O.B   Sex   Race
1._____ 2._____
3._____ 4._____

D. Involved Parties: Parents

Name (last, first, middle) *JENKINS, BILL A.* | D.O.B *6-6-59* | Sex *M* | Race *C* | Name (last, first, middle) *JENKINS, KIM P.* | D.O.B *10-11-62* | Sex *F* | Race *C*

Address *21 2nd ST., LOS ANGELES, CA* | Address *21 2nd ST., LOS ANGELES, CA*

Home Phone *(213)555-3123* Work Phone *(213)555-6644* | Home Phone *(213)555-3123* Work Phone *(213)555-7722*

E. Incident Information

IF NECESSARY, ATTACH EXTRA SHEET OR OTHER FORM AND CHECK THIS BOX ☐

1. Date/Time of Incident *1-16-94 ~7pm* | Place of Incident (check one) *HOME* ☑Occurred   ☐Observed

If child was in out-of-home care at the time of the incident, check type of care   ☐ Family Day Care
☐ Child Care Center ☐ Foster Family Home ☐ Small Family Home ☐ Group Home or Institution

2. Type of Abuse (check one):   ☑Physical ☐ Mental ☐ Sexual Assault ☐ Neglect ☐ Other

3. Narrative Description: *OBSERVED BLACK-AND-BLUE MARKS ON THE CHILD'S FOREARMS AND A CUT ABOVE HIS RIGHT EYE. CHILD SEEMED DISORIENTED, SUGGESTIVE OF CONCUSSION.*

4. Summarize what the abused child or person accompanying the child said happened:
CHILD REPORTED THAT HIS MOTHER "HURT" HIM WHEN HE SPILLED HER "WINE" AND "TALKED BACK."

5. Explain known history of similar incident(s) for this child:
No KNOWN EARLIER INCIDENTS BUT HISTORY OF ALCOHOL ABUSE BY BOTH PARENTS.

Form FPP-27-1/1-rev2/94 ©1994 GMS. Do not reproduce. For orders call (510) 865-5282, fax (510) 865-4295.

Certificate to Return to Work or School
For employer or school requirements

Over the years, I have been asked by clients to provide what is essentially an absence note for their employer or school explaining that they have been in treatment. Parents or guardians also request absence excuses for their children. The Certificate to Return to Work or School form serves this purpose nicely.

CERTIFICATE TO RETURN TO WORK OR SCHOOL

(Ms.)
Mrs.
Mr.   *MICHELLE SILVER*

has been under my care from   *9-26-92*   to   *CURRENT*

and is able to return to work/school on   *10-1-92*

Remarks: *NO RESTRICTIONS*

Clinician   *GEORGE R. JONES, Ph.D.*   Phone   *(213) 555-7927*

Address   *929 W. MAIN BLVD., STE. 101*   Date   *9-30-92*
          LOS ANGELES, CA 90000

Form FPP-28-1/1-rev2/94 ©1994 GMS. Limited permission to photocopy only. For orders call (510) 865-5282, fax (510) 865-4295.

CERTIFICATE TO RETURN TO WORK OR SCHOOL

Ms.
Mrs.
Mr.

has been under my care from   to

and is able to return to work/school on

Remarks:

Clinician   Phone

Address   Date

Form FPP-28-1/1-rev2/94 ©1994 GMS. Limited permission to photocopy only. For orders call (510) 865-5282, fax (510) 865-4295.

Fees for Depositions and Court Appearances
For statement of fees for legal consultations

My typical and usual fee for consultation in nonlegal matters is $135 per 50-minute session. Due to the nature of the legal system and the added expenses involved, such as secretarial services, record-copying services, and driving time, as well as time lost from clinical practice, it is normal to increase your fee when becoming involved in matters that concern attorneys or the court system.

The Fees for Depositions and Court Appearances form can be used to inform the agency requesting your services of your fees for such service. You can request that a minimum of 50% of the anticipated total fee be paid in advance or upon arrival at the deposition, hearing, or trial. It is important to give a copy of the form to the client also.

FEES FOR DEPOSITIONS AND COURT APPEARANCES

Date: *9-31-92*

To: *MICHELLE SILVER*

From: *GEORGE R. JONES, PH. D.*

Re: *COURT APPEARANCE- AUTO ACCIDENT*

When served with a subpoena *duces tecum* for my appearance in person or a deposition subpoena for my appearance, the following fee policies will be in effect. This is the case unless you receive a signed, written amendment from me.

My fee for scheduled appearance is $ *800.00* , paid in advance. The fee is due with the subpoena. If the fee is not paid at that time, arrangements for payment are the duty of the party requesting the appearance and must be made on receipt of this communication.

The fee is required for my scheduling the day or any fraction of the day. The fee is due whether or not I am actually called on that day. The fee is due even if the appearance is cancelled by anyone other than me for any reason and at any time. These are my usual and customary fee arrangements.

Further required attendances will be charged at additional daily rates under the same circumstances. These terms are not negotiable.

Please determine the number of days you need me, specify same, and send me a check for $ *800.00* per day by return mail if you want me to obey your subpoena. Then I will get back to you with my availability.

For payment purposes, my Federal Tax Identification Number or my Social Security Number is *999-99-9999* .

George R. Jones, Ph. D.
Signature of Clinician

Form FPP-29-1/1-rev2/94 ©1994 GMS. Limited permission to photocopy only. For orders call (510) 865-5282, fax (510) 865-4295.

Assignment of Lien
For deferment of fees for treatment, report writing, and depositions

> *lien n 1. a charge upon real or personal property for the satisfaction of some debt or duty ordinarily arising by operation of law; 2. the security interest created by a mortgage.*

Mental health practitioners are increasingly asked to act as expert witness or to prepare reports for attorneys in civil and criminal suits. Clinicians may wish to defer their fees for treatment, report writing, depositions, or other forensic-related aspects of their practice.

If you choose to provide this service for your client, the Assignment of Lien form is necessary for economic clarity between yourself, the client, and the client's legal representatives.

Before I agree to a lien, I obtain a consent to release information, then speak with the legal representatives of my client to determine the risk factors involved in collecting the fees, including the probability of collection and the potential length of time before payment will be made. I charge a higher fee for forensic work due to the fact that I may not be paid for several years and, secondarily, because I may require the services of a professional secretary for the preparation of needed reports. *Caveat:* Let the therapist beware of hidden costs when working in the legal system.

ASSIGNMENT OF LIEN

The undersigned does hereby grant to ___GEORGE R. JONES, Ph.D.___

(Clinician or Institution)

_____ for

psychological or medical services performed, a lien on any monies recovered on my behalf by way of settlement or judgment in connection with ___AUTOMOBILE ACCIDENT___

(Describe condition or incident)

_____

_____

which occurred or started on or about ___8-26-92___ .

(Date)

As of this date, ___10-4-93___ , the total amount due the provider under this lien is $ ___2000.00___
The provider of such services shall send my attorney statements for all services rendered after this date, and the lien shall be increased accordingly.

I understand that I am personally responsible for payment for all such services and that such payment is not contingent upon my receiving a settlement to a judgment.

In the event legal action is brought by the provider to enforce this lien or to receive payment for such services, the prevailing party shall be entitled to reasonable costs and attorneys fees in addition to any judgment rendered.

DATED: ___10-4-93___   CLIENT: ___Michelle Silver___

Print or type client's name: ___MICHELLE SILVER___

If the client is a minor, a parent or guardian must also sign.

PARENT or GUARDIAN: _____

The undersigned, being the attorney for the above-named client, does hereby acknowledge receipt of a copy of this Assignment of Lien and agrees to honor the lien out of any monies due to the client from any settlement or judgment.

DATED: ___10-4-93___   ATTORNEY: ___David Stein___

5

Filling in the Client's Background
Forms for Collecting Personal Information and History

This chapter discusses information gathering that will be invaluable for proceeding with psychotherapy, testifying, and report writing. The forms are printed on separate pages so that you may select the section you want to give your client to fill out at home or in the waiting room. The questions have been drawn from interviews with specialists in the fields represented, and from various questionnaires from counseling centers throughout the United States.

As we all know, asking the right question is often more important than the answer.

Confidential Personal History I and II
For compiling client information

The following forms were compiled from interviews related to the clinical treatment of mental disorders, substance-use disorders, and sexual disorders; from vocational counseling; and from report writing. These forms may be used in your practice in the preparation of reports or in direct treatment of your client.

A structured interview is sometimes antithetical to the format of psychotherapy you wish to follow. In those cases, ask your clients to complete these forms at home and advise them to circle the questions they wish to discuss in session.

These forms are extremely useful in getting a bird's-eye view of areas of your clients' lives that can reflect on their disorder and your formation of a treatment plan. You may wish to ask these questions directly because, as many clinicians voiced in the market testing of these forms, you may wish to record the affect of clients as they respond to the questions. Choose the method that is best for your clinical situation and the client you are seeing.

There are two different Confidential Personal History forms. Confidential Personal History I covers family background, health, finances, current issues, interests and traits, and educational background. It contains a section for the client to describe the events that brought her or him to your office.

Confidential Personal History II covers essentially the same areas as Personal History I. In addition, it asks about the client's religious and spiritual background, contains a check-off list of specific problem areas, inquires into the client's history of prior treatment, and includes a check-off list regarding how the client currently views her or his life.

Confidential Personal History I requires more writing; Confidential Personal History II is predominantly in a check-off format. This is important in cases where intellectual ability or writing skill may cause your client difficulty in completing one of these forms. When dealing with clients with developmental disabilities, you will probably want to ask these questions directly in a session.

CONFIDENTIAL PERSONAL HISTORY 1   (page 1 of 5)

CLIENT'S FIRST NAME: Michelle	CLIENT'S ID NO. 92-S1L-01	DATE: 9-26-92

NOTE TO CLIENT:	This personal history form is intended to help us work together. Everything is confidential. You may choose not to answer any question. Please indicate areas of particular importance to you by circling the question. Many questions can be answered by just writing "yes" or "no" or by making a check mark. Don't worry if you can't answer some of the questions, or if some do not apply to you. Just fill in the blanks as completely as you can. PLEASE PRINT OR WRITE LEGIBLY.

I. PERSONAL HISTORY

SECTION A. YOU AND YOUR FAMILY

1.	Age **34** Male (Female)
2.	How long in this state? **18 YRS.** In this country? Do you move often? **No** Seldom? **Yes**
3.	Birthplace **Portland, OR** Date of birth **9-21-92** Citizen of what nation **USA**
	Ethnic background **White**
4.	Is your ... Father living **Yes** Mother living **Yes** Together **Yes** Divorced Years divorced
5.	Was your family ... Poor (Average) Rich Language spoken at home **English**
6.	Was your home life with parents ... Unhappy (Bearable) Pleasant Very happy
7.	Is your family ... Protestant (Catholic) Jewish Other:
8.	Do you belong to a church? **No** What denomination? How often do you attend?
9.	Are you ... (Single) Engaged (No. of years) Married Widowed Separated Divorced
10.	Is your home life ... Very happy Pleasant Bearable (Unhappy)
11.	Number of brothers **5 (1 who died)** Their ages **44, 39 (Frank, dead), 36, 30**
	Number of sisters **2** Their ages **46, 38**
12.	Father's name and occupation **Anthony, bus driver**
13.	Father's abilities or special interests **Watches TV, plays card** His birthplace **Italy**
14.	Mother's name and occupation **Mary, homemaker**
15.	Mother's abilities and special interests **Cooking, sewing** Her birthplace **Italy**
16.	Father's education **12th grade** Mother's education **11th grade**
17.	What interests of your parents do you share? **Neither, except hand-work**
18.	Spouse's name **N/A** Age
19.	Spouse's work or chief interest
20.	Do you have any children? **No** Names
	Ages*

* Circle the ages of married ones

CONFIDENTIAL PERSONAL HISTORY I (page 2 of 5)

CLIENT'S FIRST NAME: Michelle	CLIENT'S ID NO. 92-SIL-01	DATE: 9-26-92

SECTION B. YOUR HEALTH

1. Height 5' 8" Weight 135 Physical condition: Excellent Good Fair (Poor)

2. Please describe any physical handicaps or health worries that bother you. I have not feeling well since the car accident (August 26). I have been having nightmares and sleep poorly. I feel dizzy at times.

3. What do you do to keep in good physical condition? Nothing

4. Are you able to relax easily after strenuous effort? No   Are you happy most of the time? No

5. What worries, anxieties, or strong prejudices do you have? Worried about my job. My boss yells at us a lot. He is angry about the car accident.

6. When was your last complete physical examination? 2-1-92 What was the result? Results OK

7. When did you last visit a doctor? 8-28-92 Why? Car accident

8. Have you ever been refused insurance or employment because of a physical or psychological condition? No

   If so, please explain.

SECTION C. YOUR FINANCES

1. Do you have an independent income? Yes   Do you have a system of saving money? Yes

   Are you currently in financial crisis? Not really

2. How many dependents do you have? None   Their ages

   Relationship to you?

3. What financial help are you seeking in order to carry out your educational, vocational, or other plans?

4. If you do not pay your bills, who assists you?

II. YOUR ISSUES

1. Briefly describe the issues that are important to you. Please mention any ambitions, difficulties, obstacles, etc., even if they seem relatively unimportant.

   My career. It's important that I support myself. and sometimes help my parents.
   I wanted to become an accountant in a company. So I went to Business School and got a Certificate. My parents were not interested in my going to school for more education. They thought I should become a dress-maker like my sister.

CONFIDENTIAL PERSONAL HISTORY I (page 3 of 5)

CLIENT'S FIRST NAME: Michelle	CLIENT'S ID NO. 92-SIC-01	DATE: 9-26-92

2. How long have these issues been important? 20 YRS.   What avenues have you explored to work on them? Career counseling w/ George Jones

3. Have you consulted anyone professionally about these issues? **YES**   If so, whom? You

4. With whom do you usually talk over your problems or plans? Best friend, Ruth

5. In what ways is your family sympathetic or unsympathetic toward your issues?

My parents want me to marry and have a family like my sister.

6. Do you have any special dreams or goals that currently influence you?

I never want to spend my time at work standing. I want a career where I can move about the city or sit at my desk.

III. YOUR INTERESTS AND TRAITS

1. What are your present hobbies or keen interests? Cross-stitch, hand-work, crafts.

2. Past hobbies or interests (if different)? Sketching and drawing.

3. To what clubs and organizations do you now belong? Accountants' Association

4. Is your social activity chiefly with groups of your own age? **YES** Older? **No** Younger? **No**

5. In what activities have you taken a leading role? Sec'y - Accountant's Association

6. For what activities do you wish you had more money or time? I would like to travel around this country and other countries.

7. In sports, would you rather be a player or a spectator? Spectator

8. What do you enjoy more than anything else? Eating

9. What habits do you have that might hinder your greater success? I over-organize

10. What sort of person do you like best? Someone organized and who is "together."

11. What kind of person do you dislike? Anyone who is angry and yells at me.

12. Do you have many acquaintances? Some   How many close friends? One

13. Do you have feelings of failure? Yes   If so, about what? My job. Am I going to be fired?

14. In what ways, if any, do you lack confidence in yourself? I thought I was doing a good job.

15. In the spaces below, list four or five of your prominent character traits:

a. Strengths	b. Weaknesses
Good at organizing Feel responsible in my work. I work hard.	I'll work overtime for no extra pay. I don't feel physically strong now. I try to handle more than my share of the work.

CONFIDENTIAL PERSONAL HISTORY I   (page 4 of 5)

CLIENT'S FIRST NAME: Michelle	CLIENT'S ID NO. 92-SIL-01	DATE: 9-26-92

IV. YOUR EDUCATION

1. List schools and colleges attended. (Name last one first)

Name	Dates	Grade completed or degree
Business College	1986	Accounting Certificate
El Camino College	1978	60 units
Los Angeles H.S.	1976	Diploma

2. How well did you like school? It was O.K.

3. If starting over, would you choose the same line of study? Yes

4. What magazines do you subscribe to? PROFESSIONAL ACCOUNTING, TIME, NEWSWEEK

5. If your education has been (or may be) cut off before completion, why? Yes. Couldn't work and attend school at the same time.

6. What further education do you plan? Complete college degree, maybe

7. List studies that you like very much: Literature, History, Music

8. List those you dislike: Physical Education, languages.

9. Has school been: easy   (fairly easy)   difficult   very difficult

10. What training or courses taken do you consider most valuable to you? Accounting classes

11. In what fields of learning are you best informed? Accounting

12. In what extracurricular activities have you been active? Sang in the choir

13. What achievements in school gave (or give) you great satisfaction? Enjoyed being in the choir. My A+ in History.

14. If you had the time, what books would you like to read? I love romances, historical novels.

15. Of books you have read, did any make a great impression on you? If so, which? I think 'gone with the Wind' is the best book I've read.

16. What traveling have you done, and what about it greatly impressed you? I haven't done a lot of traveling. Just Portland to Los Angeles. I would like to travel more around the States.

CONFIDENTIAL PERSONAL HISTORY I   (page 5 of 5)

CLIENT'S FIRST NAME: Michelle	CLIENT'S ID NO. 92-SIL-01	DATE: 9-26-92

V. YOUR STORY

In the space below, write anything you wish to tell about your life that you think is important. Especially describe the events that gave you great joy or great disappointment.

Life in Oregon — I was born in Portland. Both my parents worked. Everyone was expected to work from early on. My sister already had a craft — sewing. I ran errands and had a paper-route.

Coming to California. — We came to LA. It was an opportunity for a better life. My parents had friends here. But we kids didn't know anyone.

Working as nurse's aide — Was not a very good job. I hated being on my feet as much each day. My goal was a job where I could sit. But I didn't want to make clothes like my sister. There was something better to do.

School — I wanted more education. My parents didn't encourage me. They wanted me to work like my sister. Girls didn't need so much education — it is mostly for the sons. But they were happy when I started bringing in good money — more than ever before. That was satisfying.

Car accidents — My boss was always yelling at me. And sending me on errands for his private business. While I was doing that one day I had a terrible accident. He was abusive about the accident and the fact I couldn't complete his errands.

CONFIDENTIAL PERSONAL HISTORY II   (page 1 of 8)

CLIENT'S FIRST NAME: Michelle	CLIENT'S ID NO. 92-SIL-01	DATE: 9-26-92

SECTION I. YOU AND YOUR FAMILY

1.	Sex: Male (Female) Age: 34 Birthday (Month-Day-Year): 9-21-58				
2.	What ethnicity do you consider yourself, other than American? Italian				
3.	Your place of birth: Portland, OR Where did you grow up? Portland, L.A.				
4.	How many times in the past year did you change residence? None Past 2 years Once				
	Past 3 years Twice Past 5 years Twice Past 10 years Three Past 20 years Three				
5.	Which parent was more interested in you? Both				
6.	In which parent were you more interested? Mother				
7.	Your marital status: (Single) Married Age married: You Your spouse				
8.	Number of children: Girls/ ages None Boys/ ages None				

9.	History of divorce or separation in your family	No	Yes	Times	Your age
	Paternal grandparents	✓			
	Maternal grandparents	✓			
	Father	✓			
	Mother	✓			
	You	✓			

10.	If divorced, did your parents remarry? Mother Father		
11.	Is your parents' marriage a marriage of mixed ethnicity? (No) Yes		
	Of what ethnic groups?		
12.	Do you consider your marriage a marriage of mixed ethnicity? No Yes		
	Of what ethnic groups?		
13.	Were you an adopted child? Yes (No)		
14.	If yes, do you have feelings about this? None at all Very few Definite Extreme		
15.	If yes, at what age were you told you were an adopted child?		
16.	Were you a wanted child? (Yes) No		
17.	Do you have feelings about this? None at all Very few (Definite) Extreme		
18.	During your upbringing, how many dependents was the family breadwinner responsible for? 9		

Form FPP-32-1/8-rev2/94 ©1994 GMS. Limited permission to photocopy only. For orders call (510) 865-5282, fax (510) 865-4295.

CONFIDENTIAL PERSONAL HISTORY II   (page 2 of 8)

CLIENT'S FIRST NAME: Michelle	CLIENT'S ID NO. 92-51L-01	DATE: 9-26-92

SECTION II. HEALTH

1. Height: 5' 8"   Weight: 170   Physical condition: Excellent   Good   Fair   (Poor)

2. When was your last complete physical examination? (Approximate date—month and year) 2/92

3. Are you presently under a doctor's care for any condition?   Yes   (No)

    If yes, name condition:

4. List your doctor's diagnoses of acute or chronic disease, disabling or not:

5. Are you presently taking any medications: Yes   (No)

    If yes, list medications and dosages:

6. Please list types and dates of major surgical operations: Gall bladder surgery in 1980. Foot surgery in 1984.

7. Do you have a physical disability? No   If yes, type of disability:

8. Have you been refused insurance or employment because of your physical condition?   Yes   (No)

9. Have you been hospitalized for chemical abuse?   Yes   (No)

10. Have you ever been hospitalized for chemical abuse but diagnosed as having something else (including a fracture)?   Yes   (No)

    Diagnosis:

11. Do you have a physical fitness program?   (Not at all)   Occasionally   Regularly (2–3 times a week)

12. Do you presently experience severe emotional and mood changes to the point where they make it difficult to function at your normal level: Never   Seldom   (Often (6 times a year))

    Circle which kind(s):   (Anxiety)   (Frustration)   Manic states   (Depression)

13. As a child did you experience enuresis (bed wetting)?   Never   Seldom ✓   Often

14. How was your home life as a child?   (Unhappy)   Bearable   Pleasant   Very happy

15. How is your home life presently?   (Unhappy)   Bearable   Pleasant   Very happy

16. Is your father alive?   (Yes)   No

    If not, what was the cause of his death?   How old were you?

17. Is your mother alive?   (Yes)   No

    If not, what was the cause of her death?   How old were you?

Form FPP-32-2/8-rev2/94 ©1994 GMS. Limited permission to photocopy only. For orders call (510) 865-5282, fax (510) 865-4295.

CONFIDENTIAL PERSONAL HISTORY II (page 3 of 8)

CLIENT'S FIRST NAME: Michelle	CLIENT'S ID NO. 92-512-01	DATE: 9-26-92

SECTION III. SPIRITUALITY

		Not at all	Possibly	Definitely
1.	Do you believe in God or a Higher Power?			✓
2.	Are you agnostic? (believe you can't know about God)	✓		
3.	Are you atheistic? (believe God does not exist)	✓		
4.	Are you antireligious or antispiritual?	✓		
5.	In the past, did you believe in God or a Higher Power?			✓
6.	In the past, were you agnostic?	✓		
7.	In the past, were you atheistic?	✓		
8.	In the past, were you antireligious or antispiritual?		✓	
9.	The name of your spiritual program or religion, if structured or formal: Roman Catholic			
10.	The name of your spiritual program or group, if unstructured or informal:			

		Not at all	Occasionally	Regularly
11.	Do you attend religious activities?	✓		
12.	Did you attend religious activities as a child?			✓
13.	What was the religious background of your parents? Catholic Name of religion: Catholicism			

		Not at all	Occasionally	Regularly
14.	Do your parents attend religious activities?			✓
15.	In the past, did your parents attend religious activities?			✓

SECTION IV. FINANCES

		Poor	Lower middle	Upper middle	Rich
1.	Describe your parents' standard of living:		✓		
2.	Describe your standard of living:		✓		

3.	Do you have an independent income?	(Yes)	No		
4.	Do you have a system of saving money?	(Yes)	No		
5.	How often do you withdraw from your savings?	Not at all	Seldom	(Frequently)	Regularly
6.	Are you in financial crisis?	(Yes)	No		
7.	Number of dependents: Spouse	Children	Parents	Grandparents	
	Brothers	Sisters	Uncles	Aunts	Others:
8.	Do you need financial help to complete educational, vocational, or other plans?	Yes	(No)		
9.	Do you pay your own bills?	(All)	Most	Few	None
10.	Your annual income: Under $10,000	$10–20,000	($20–30,000)	$30–50,000	$50,000+ $100,000+
11.	Do you live comfortably on your income?	(Yes)	No		
12.	Do you think other people could live comfortably on your income?	(Yes)	No		
13.	How much income would satisfy you now? $ 30,000 10 years from now? $ 75,000				

Form FPP-32-3/8-rev2/94 ©1994 GMS. Limited permission to photocopy only. For orders call (510) 865-5282, fax (510) 865-4295.

CONFIDENTIAL PERSONAL HISTORY II   (page 4 of 8)

CLIENT'S FIRST NAME: Michelle	CLIENT'S ID NO. 92-SIL-01	DATE: 9-26-92

SECTION V. EDUCATION

1. How many years have you been registered full-time in school? **13**
2. How many years have you been registered part-time in school? **2**
3. How may degrees have you received? (High school)   B.A. or B.S.   M.A. or M.S.   Ph.D.

   Other professional degrees: **Accounting Certificate**

4. Indicate your scholastic standing. If you used alcohol or drugs, did it help or hinder your scholastic standing?

Scholastic standing:	High	Medium	Low	Helped	Hindered
High school		✓			
B.A. or B.S.					
M.A. or M.S.					
Ph.D.					
Other professional degrees	✓				

5. In the past two years, how many hours of continuing education have you completed? **None**

6. Do you habitually read magazines? (Yes)   No
7. Do you habitually read books? (Yes)   No
8. Do you read to further your education?   For pleasure?   To escape?   All three? **Yes**
9. Are you interested in furthering your education? (Yes)   No
10. Has school study been easy? **Fairly easy**

		Not at all	Slightly	Definitely	Extremely
11.	Do you feel your intelligence is below that of other people?	✓			
12.	Do you feel your intelligence is above that of other people?			✓	
13.	Do you feel your education is below that of other people?		✓		
14.	Do you feel your education is above that of other people?	✓			
15.	Do you feel your intelligence level is superior to your education level?			✓	
16.	Do you feel your education level is superior to your intelligence level?	✓			

CONFIDENTIAL PERSONAL HISTORY II (page 5 of 8)				
CLIENT'S FIRST NAME: Michelle	CLIENT'S ID NO. 92-SIL-01		DATE: 9-26-92	

SECTION VI. PROBLEM AREAS

	I. Which of the following people are or were sources of anxiety or frustration:	None	Mild	Definite	Extreme
a.	paternal grandfather, presently	✓			
	paternal grandfather, in the past	✓			
b.	paternal grandmother, presently	✓			
	paternal grandmother, in the past	✓			
c.	maternal grandfather, presently	✓			
	maternal grandfather, in the past	✓			
d.	maternal grandmother, presently	✓			
	maternal grandmother, in the past	✓			
e.	father, presently			✓	
	father, in the past				✓
f.	mother, presently		✓		
	mother, in the past		✓		
g.	brothers, presently	✓			
	brothers, in the past			✓	
h.	sisters, presently			✓	
	sisters, in the past		✓		
i.	spouse or lover, presently				
	spouse or lover, in the past				
j.	sons, presently				
	sons, in the past				
k.	daughters, presently				
	daughters, in the past				
l.	supervisor, presently				✓
	supervisor, in the past				✓
m.	fellow workers, peers, male, presently	✓			
	fellow workers, peers, male, in the past	✓			
n.	fellow workers, peers, female, presently	✓			
	fellow workers, peers, female, in the past	✓			
o.	friends, male, presently		✓		
	friends, male, in the past		✓		
p.	friends, female, presently	✓			
	friends, female, in the past	✓			

Form FPP-32-5/8-rev2/94 ©1994 GMS. Limited permission to photocopy only. For orders call (510) 865-5282, fax (510) 865-4295.

CONFIDENTIAL PERSONAL HISTORY II (page 6 of 8)

CLIENT'S FIRST NAME: Michelle	CLIENT'S ID NO. 92-512-01	DATE: 9-26-92

	SECTION VI. (CONTINUED)	None	Mild	Definite	Extreme
2.	If you consider yourself a professional, is working with nonprofessionals a source of anxiety?		✓		
3.	If you are a nonprofessional, is working with professionals a source of anxiety?				
4.	If you have had a life experience of chemical abuse (addiction or alcoholism), is working with people who have not experienced addiction or alcoholism a source of anxiety?				
5.	If you have not had a life experience of chemical abuse (addiction or alcoholism), is working with people who have experienced addiction or alcoholism a source of anxiety?			✓	
6.	Check fears or phobias below:				
a.	heights	✓			
b.	closed areas	✓			
c.	dark	✓			
d.	animals	✓			
e.	opposite sex		✓		
f.	people	✓			
g.	driving			✓	
h.	water	✓			
i.	fire			✓	
j.	being touched		✓		
k.	own death			✓	
l.	other's death			✓	
m.	flying	✓			
n.	travel	✓			
o.	other:				

7.	Have you sought help for any of your problems? Yes (No)
	If yes, in what way?
a.	Self-help, 12-step, or other programs (AA, Al-Anon, Narcotics Anonymous, etc.)
	Name: Success:
b.	Professional (psychiatrist, psychologist, social worker, counselor, minister, priest, rabbi, etc.)
	Type: Success:
c.	Nonprofessional (church, spiritual source including spiritual groups or organizations)
	Name: Success:
d.	Other source (specify):
	Success:

Form FPP-32-6/8-rev2/94 ©1994 GMS. Limited permission to photocopy only. For orders call (510) 865-5282, fax (510) 865-4295.

CONFIDENTIAL PERSONAL HISTORY II　(page 7 of 8)

CLIENT'S FIRST NAME: Michelle	CLIENT'S ID NO. 92-51L-01	DATE: 9-26-92

	SECTION VI. (CONTINUED)	None	One	2–5	6–10	Over 10
8.	How many meaningful persons are in your life to whom you feel committed and with whom you share yourself totally?			✓		
9.	How many meaningful persons are in your life with whom you would share almost anything?			✓		
10.	How many people in your life do you feel are simply "close friends"?			✓		
11.	How many people are in your life whom you are not close to but whom you feel comfortable being around?				✓	

12.	Have you found it difficult to find a suitable mate?　Yes　(No)
13.	If you have been able to find a suitable mate or mates, have you found it difficult to maintain a meaningful relationship?　(Yes)　No
14.	Have you been able to find a suitable mate and maintain a meaningful relationship?　Yes　(No)

		No	Mild	Definite	Extreme
15.	Do you feel you lack self-control and discipline?	✓			
16.	Do you feel you lack self-confidence?		✓		
17.	Do you feel self-conscious or shy in groups?			✓	
18.	Do you feel you lack meaningful goals?		✓		
19.	Do you feel you live your life satisfying other people's goals?			✓	
20.	Do you feel most of your friends dominate you?		✓		
21.	Do you feel you dominate most of your friends?	✓			
22.	Do you feel unable to accept affection?	✓			
23.	Do you feel unable to give affection?	✓			
24.	Do you feel you are a compulsive person?		✓		
25.	Do you feel you are an intolerant person?	✓			
26.	Do you feel you are an impatient person?		✓		
27.	Do you feel you demand too much perfection from yourself?		✓		
28.	Do you feel there is a lack of communication between you and other people?			✓	

CONFIDENTIAL PERSONAL HISTORY II   (page 8 of 8)

CLIENT'S FIRST NAME: **Michelle**   CLIENT'S ID NO. **92-51L-01**   DATE: **9-26-92**

	SECTION VI. (CONTINUED)	Never	Seldom	Frequently	Regularly
29.	Have you ever had suicidal thoughts?			✓	
30.	Have you ever had suicidal dreams?			✓	
31.	Have you ever made definite suicidal plans?		✓		
32.	Have you ever attempted suicide?	✓			
33.	Have you been aware of causing a crisis as a way of asking for help?	✓			

Confidential Vocational History
For evaluating past and present levels of functioning

This questionnaire is particularly useful in helping to understand Axis V levels of functioning (GAF scales of the DSM) in the client's past and present. This form will help you investigate clients' expectations regarding their vocational and economic future. It will help you spot significant traumatic events the client may be unaware of that have significantly changed her or his level of functioning. It also aids in reality-testing your client's expectations of herself or himself, and of others.

CONFIDENTIAL VOCATIONAL HISTORY (page 1 of 4)

CLIENT'S FIRST NAME: Michelle	CLIENT'S ID. NO: 92-51L-01	DATE: 9-26-92

SECTION A. EXPERIENCE

1. Present occupation: Bookkeeper   Do you like it? Yes   How long in this job? 21 mos

   Describe what you do: Accounting, keep financial records

2. How many years have you been working? 19   How many positions? 5   Soc. Security No. 222-22-2222

3. List work you have done. Include part-time and any government or armed service jobs. Put present job first.

Your job or position	Date began and left	Weekly wage	Why left?
E&M Computers	Jan '91 to now	$ 425.00	
Electronics Co.	1990 - 1991	$ 400.00	Out of business
ADS Management	1985 - 1990	$ 400.00	Better job
St. Mary's hospital	1976 - 1985	$ 350.00	Better job
St. Mary's - training	1974 - 1976		

(Attach extra sheet if you need more space)

4. Which work did you like best? Electronics Co.   Why? Nice people

5. In what way have you been dissatisfied with any job you have held? Nurse's aide. Didn't pay enough to be on my feet all day.

6. Do you have any difficulty in getting a job when unemployed?

7. Have you any type of occupational license? No   Do you belong to a union? No

SECTION B. INFORMATION

1. What recent reading have you done that gave you occupational information?
   Wall Street Journal, Accountants' Assn Magazine

2. For what type of work are you fitted now? Accountant / Bookkeeper

3. List the general occupational fields about which you would like to learn more:
   Computers (to keep up with Accounting Field)

4. What career has been suggested often for you? Accounting / Travel Agent

5. What vocation do (or did) your parents want you to follow? Dress-making

6. What family or other conditions affected your vocational choice? Had to go against the advice of my family to go to school and into accounting

7. In what occupations are some of your close relatives very successful?
   Brother is a computer programmer; sister styles clothes.

CONFIDENTIAL VOCATIONAL HISTORY (page 2 of 4)

CLIENT'S FIRST NAME: Michelle	CLIENT'S ID NO. 92-SIL-01	DATE: 9-26-92

SECTION C. APTITUDES AND PREFERENCES

1. What are your greatest vocational assets (qualities, special abilities, skills, etc.)?
I'm careful and diligent.
I like working with figures. I want to improve myself.

2. If you could choose now, without any financial restrictions, the occupation in which you would like to be engaged 10 years from now, what would it be? Designing Accounting Systems

3. How long have you had this ambition? 4 YRS. Do you feel blocked? Yes

4. What sorts of work have you thought you might enjoy (even if you have not tried them)?
Computer Programming. Travel Agent

5. List three to six occupations in which you think you could be reasonably happy, in order of preference.

a. Accounting System Design	d.
b. Accountant - Large Firm	e.
c. Accountant - Small Firm	f.

6. Have you planned a career? Yes   If so, what? Towards Systems Design

7. How have you planned to reach this goal? More education.

SECTION D. JOBS AND HOBBIES

Look over these lists and circle the jobs or hobbies that fit your experience. If you have spent time in jobs or hobbies not included, enter them under the appropriate headings on this and the following page.

1. PRIMARILY EGO-SATISFYING	2. RESCUING PEOPLE	3. MANAGING PEOPLE	4. HELPING PEOPLE
a. actor	a. counselor	(a.) administrator	a. beautician
b. animal trainer	b. doctor	b. chairperson	b. clerk
c. dangerous jobs	c. firefighter	c. coach	c. interpreter
d. diver	d. minister	d. department store owner-manager	d. librarian
e. explorer	e. nurse	e. executive	e. receptionist
f. mountain climber	f. occupation therapist	f. politician	f. salesperson
(g.) musician	g. physical therapist	g. president	g. secretary
h. athlete	h. priest	h. school principal	h. taxi driver
i.	i. psychiatrist	i. supervisor	i. teacher
j.	j. psychologist	j.	(j.) waiter / waitress
k.	k. rabbi	k.	k. bartender
	l. social worker	l.	l.
	m. speech therapist		m.
	n. veterinarian		n.
	o. nurse's aide		
	p.		
	q.		

Form FPP-33-2/4-rev2/94 ©1994 GMS. Limited permission to photocopy only. For orders call (510) 865-5282, fax (510) 865-4295.

CONFIDENTIAL VOCATIONAL HISTORY   (page 3 of 4)

CLIENT'S FIRST NAME: Michelle	CLIENT'S ID NO. 92-51L-01	DATE: 9-26-92

5. MANAGING (NONPEOPLE)	6. TECHNICAL TRADES	7. SEMITECHNICAL SERVICES	10. NONTECHNICAL SERVICES
a. control clerk	a. builder	a. assembly line worker	a. gas station operator
b. inventory clerk	b. broker	b. bricklayer	b. hard laborer
c. office manager	c. chemist	c. carpenter	c. machine operator
d. project manager	d. engineer	d. construction worker	d.
e. purchasing agent	e. pharmacist	e. dental technician	e.
f. **Bookkeeper**	f. research analyst	f. file clerk	f.
g.	g. research specialist	g. gardener	
h.	h. **Accountant**	h. purchasing agent	
	i.	i. repairperson	
	j.	j.	
		k.	
		l.	

9. ENFORCEMENT SERVICES	10. MISCELLANEOUS	11. SOCIALLY DISAPPROVED
a. bill collector	a. housewife/husband	a. hustler
b. FBI agent	b. student	b. drug dealer
c. guard	c. unemployed	c. drug smuggler
d. IRS agent	d.	d. pimp / madame
e. investigator	e.	e. prostitute / gigolo
f. parole agent	f.	f. thief
g. police officer		g.
h.		h.
i.		i.
j.		

		First	Second	Third
1.	Of those jobs you have done, which have been the most enjoyable? List them in order of preference.	Accountant	Bookkeeper	Nurse's Aide
2.	How long have you worked in each job listed for question 1? (years and months)	3 YEARS	3 YEARS	9 YEARS
3.	List, in order of preference, the hobbies you have had that have been the most enjoyable.	Cooking	Music	Hand-work
4.	How long have you participated in each hobby listed for question 3? (years and months)	19 YEARS	3 YEARS	20 YEARS
5.	List, in order of preference, the jobs you haven't done but would like to try.	Computer Programming	System Design	Supervisor
6.	List, in order of preference, the hobbies you haven't had but would like to try.	Painting	Ice-Skating	Skiing
7.	List those jobs or hobbies you have done that were the most distasteful.	Waitress	Laundry	Cleaning

CONFIDENTIAL VOCATIONAL HISTORY　(page 4 of 4)

CLIENT'S FIRST NAME: Michelle	CLIENT'S ID NO. 92-51L-01	DATE: 9-26-92

		First	Second	Third
8.	Of those jobs or hobbies you haven't done, which would be most distasteful?	House-Keeper		
9.	What jobs or hobbies would you consider only if the pay-off in satisfaction or salary were right?	House-wife		
10.	What jobs or hobbies would you not consider under any circumstances?	Gardening	Go-Go Dancer	File clerk
11.	If it could be kept absolutely secret, what jobs or hobbies would you consider trying?	Ice dancing	Yoga	Write a book

12.	What jobs or hobbies were you coerced into doing to please someone else? Explain.
	Waitress. Jobs were easy for me to get. Could bring momey into the family.

13.	What jobs or hobbies have others tried to coerce you out of pursuing? Explain.
	Accounting. Family thought it was a man's job.

Form FPP-33-4/4-rev2/94 ©1994 GMS. Limited permission to photocopy only. For orders call (510) 865-5282, fax (510) 865-4295.

Confidential Chemical (Substance Use) History
For evaluation of chemical use

The Confidential Chemical (Substance Use) History form is helpful for evaluating the history and extent of a client's use of chemicals. By requiring the client to divide her or his life into three periods based on her or his substance-use history, this form helps you understand the development of the client's chemical dependency. It also helps you understand how the client perceives changes, if any, that could be correlated to chemical use. I have found that clients are very adept at seeing their own phases of substance use. You may wish to explore with your clients the psychosocial stressors that were present at the time of changes in substance use.

The final section of the Confidential Chemical History is the substance-use history of the clients' significant others, which is extremely useful information rarely covered in other forms. This clinical information may help you in determining sociological, psychological, biological, or hereditary trends in your client's history.

CONFIDENTIAL CHEMICAL (SUBSTANCE USE) HISTORY   (page 1 of 13)

CLIENT'S FIRST NAME: Michelle	CLIENT'S ID NO. 92-512-01	DATE: 9-30-92

This is a four-part questionnaire. The first three parts are for you to divide your substance use into three periods: A. EARLY PERIOD, B. MIDDLE PERIOD, and C. LATER PERIOD. The fourth part, D, is for recording the substance use history of your significant others. Please check all questions, even when substance use is similar in all periods. Please include nonprescription and prescription medications that affect your mood.

A. EARLY PERIOD

		Never	1–4 times a year	5–12 times a year	2–7 times a month	2–4 times a week	5–7 times a week	Several times a day
1.	How many years does this period cover:							
2.	Your age at the start of this period:							
3.	How often did you use:							
	a. Alcohol (wine)				✓			
	b. Nicotine	✓						
	c. Caffeine					✓		
	d. Marijuana, euphoriants	✓						
	e. Stimulants, cocaine, amphetamines	✓						
	f. Depressants, tranquilizers, painkillers	✓						
	g. Hallucinogens, LSD, mushrooms, peyote, PCP	✓						
	h. Narcotics, barbiturates, other	✓						

4.	What was your maximum daily dose during your heaviest use of:	
	a. Alcohol 1 glass	b. Nicotine
	c. Caffeine 2 cups	d. Marijuana, euphoriants
	e. Stimulants, cocaine, amphetamines	f. Depressants, tranquilizers, painkillers
	g. Hallucinogens, etc.	h. Narcotics, barbiturates, other

5.	How many physical disabilities due to your use of:	None	1	2–5	6–10	10 +
	a. Alcohol	✓				
	b. Nicotine	✓				
	c. Caffeine	✓				
	d. Marijuana, euphoriants	✓				
	e. Stimulants, cocaine, amphetamines	✓				
	f. Depressants, tranquilizers, painkillers	✓				
	g. Hallucinogens, LSD, mushrooms, peyote, PCP	✓				
	h. Narcotics, barbiturates, other	✓				

Form FPP-34-1/13-rev2/94 ©1994 GMS. Limited permission to photocopy only. For orders call (510) 865-5282, fax (510) 865-4295.

CONFIDENTIAL CHEMICAL (SUBSTANCE USE) HISTORY   (page 2 of 13)
A. EARLY PERIOD (CONTINUED)

CLIENT'S FIRST NAME: Michelle   CLIENT'S ID NO. 92-5 IL-01   DATE: 9-30-92

	None	1	2–5	6–10	10+
6. How many hospitalizations due to your use of:					
a. Alcohol	✓				
b. Nicotine	✓				
c. Caffeine	✓				
d. Marijuana, euphoriants	✓				
e. Stimulants, cocaine, amphetamines	✓				
f. Depressants, tranquilizers, painkillers	✓				
g. Hallucinogens, LSD, mushrooms, peyote, PCP	✓				
h. Narcotics, barbiturates, other	✓				
7. How many arrests while driving have you had due to your use of:					
a. Alcohol	✓				
b. Nicotine	✓				
c. Caffeine	✓				
d. Marijuana, euphoriants	✓				
e. Stimulants, cocaine, amphetamines	✓				
f. Depressants, tranquilizers, painkillers	✓				
g. Hallucinogens, LSD, mushrooms, peyote, PCP	✓				
h. Narcotics, barbiturates, other	✓				
8. How many times have you lost your driver's license due to the use of:					
a. Alcohol	✓				
b. Nicotine	✓				
c. Caffeine	✓				
d. Marijuana, euphoriants	✓				
e. Stimulants, cocaine, amphetamines	✓				
f. Depressants, tranquilizers, painkillers	✓				
g. Hallucinogens, LSD, mushrooms, peyote, PCP	✓				
h. Narcotics, barbiturates, other	✓				
9. How many nondriving arrests due to the use of:					
a. Alcohol	✓				
b. Nicotine	✓				
c. Caffeine	✓				
d. Marijuana, euphoriants	✓				
e. Stimulants, cocaine, amphetamines	✓				
f. Depressants, tranquilizers, painkillers	✓				
g. Hallucinogens, LSD, mushrooms, peyote, PCP	✓				
h. Narcotics, barbiturates, other	✓				

CONFIDENTIAL CHEMICAL (SUBSTANCE USE) HISTORY   (page 3 of 13)
A. EARLY PERIOD (CONTINUED)

CLIENT'S FIRST NAME: Michelle	CLIENT'S ID NO. 92-SIL-01	DATE: 9-30-92

	None	1	2–5	6–10	10 +
10. How many arrests for violence due to the use of:					
a. Alcohol	✓				
b. Nicotine	✓				
c. Caffeine	✓				
d. Marijuana, euphoriants	✓				
e. Stimulants, cocaine, amphetamines	✓				
f. Depressants, tranquilizers, painkillers	✓				
g. Hallucinogens, LSD, mushrooms, peyote, PCP	✓				
h. Narcotics, barbiturates, other	✓				
11. How many ticket citations have you received while under the influence of:					
a. Alcohol	✓				
b. Nicotine	✓				
c. Caffeine	✓				
d. Marijuana, euphoriants	✓				
e. Stimulants, cocaine, amphetamines	✓				
f. Depressants, tranquilizers, painkillers	✓				
g. Hallucinogens, LSD, mushrooms, peyote, PCP	✓				
h. Narcotics, barbiturates, other	✓				
12. How many tickets have you received while NOT under the influence of:					
Alcohol, depressants, stimulants, marijuana, hallucinogens or narcotics?	✓				
13. How many times have you been stopped by the police but not arrested while under the influence of:					
a. Alcohol	✓				
b. Nicotine	✓				
c. Caffeine	✓				
d. Marijuana, euphoriants	✓				
e. Stimulants, cocaine, amphetamines	✓				
f. Depressants, tranquilizers, painkillers	✓				
g. Hallucinogens, LSD, mushrooms, peyote, PCP	✓				
h. Narcotics, barbiturates, other	✓				

Form FPP-34-3/13-rev2/94 ©1994 GMS. Limited permission to photocopy only. For orders call (510) 865-5282, fax (510) 865-4295.

CONFIDENTIAL CHEMICAL (SUBSTANCE USE) HISTORY (page 4 of 13)
A. EARLY PERIOD (CONTINUED)

CLIENT'S FIRST NAME: Michelle	CLIENT'S ID NO. 92-51L-01		DATE: 9-30-92		
	None	1	2–5	6–10	10 +
14. How many times did you miss work as a result of the use of:					
a. Alcohol	✓				
b. Nicotine	✓				
c. Caffeine	✓				
d. Marijuana, euphoriants	✓				
e. Stimulants, cocaine, amphetamines	✓				
f. Depressants, tranquilizers, painkillers	✓				
g. Hallucinogens, LSD, mushrooms, peyote, PCP	✓				
h. Narcotics, barbiturates, other	✓				
15. How many times did you lose or change jobs as a result of the use of:					
a. Alcohol	✓				
b. Nicotine	✓				
c. Caffeine	✓				
d. Marijuana, euphoriants	✓				
e. Stimulants, cocaine, amphetamines	✓				
f. Depressants, tranquilizers, painkillers	✓				
g. Hallucinogens, LSD, mushrooms, peyote, PCP	✓				
h. Narcotics, barbiturates, other	✓				
16. How many times have you been separated or divorced from spouse or loved one due to the use of:					
a. Alcohol	✓				
b. Nicotine	✓				
c. Caffeine	✓				
d. Marijuana, euphoriants	✓				
e. Stimulants, cocaine, amphetamines	✓				
f. Depressants, tranquilizers, painkillers	✓				
g. Hallucinogens, LSD, mushrooms, peyote, PCP	✓				
h. Narcotics, barbiturates, other	✓				
17. In your opinion, did your abuse of chemicals interfere with the style of life you wanted to lead?	(Not at all)	Mildly		Definitely	Extremely

Form FPP-34-4/13-rev2/94 ©1994 GMS. Limited permission to photocopy only. For orders call (510) 865-5282, fax (510) 865-4295.

CONFIDENTIAL CHEMICAL (SUBSTANCE USE) HISTORY (page 5 of 13)

CLIENT'S FIRST NAME: Michelle	CLIENT'S ID NO. 92·512-01	DATE: 9-30-92

Please answer the questions as they relate to the middle period of your substance use. Check all questions, even when substance use is similar in all periods. Please include nonprescription and prescription medications that affect your mood.

B. MIDDLE PERIOD

		Never	1–4 times a year	5–12 times a year	2–7 times a month	2–4 times a week	5–7 times a week	Several times a day
1.	How many years does this period cover: 7							
2.	Your age at the start of this period: 21							
3.	How often did you use:							
	a. Alcohol				✓			
	b. Nicotine	✓						
	c. Caffeine						✓	
	d. Marijuana, euphoriants		✓					
	e. Stimulants, cocaine, amphetamines			✓				
	f. Depressants, tranquilizers, painkillers	✓						
	g. Hallucinogens, LSD, mushrooms, peyote, PCP	✓						
	h. Narcotics, barbiturates, other	✓						

4.	What was your maximum daily dose during your heaviest use of:		
	a. Alcohol 2 glasses of wine	b. Nicotine	
	c. Caffeine	d. Marijuana, euphoriants 2 joints	
	e. Stimulants, cocaine, amphetamines 3 lines	f. Depressants, tranquilizers, painkillers	
	g. Hallucinogens, etc.	h. Narcotics, barbiturates, other	

5.	How many physical disabilities due to the use of:	None	One	2–5	6–10	10 +
	a. Alcohol	✓				
	b. Nicotine	✓				
	c. Caffeine	✓				
	d. Marijuana, euphoriants	✓				
	e. Stimulants, cocaine, amphetamines	✓				
	f. Depressants, tranquilizers, painkillers	✓				
	g. Hallucinogens, LSD, mushrooms, peyote, PCP	✓				
	h. Narcotics, barbiturates, other	✓				

CONFIDENTIAL CHEMICAL (SUBSTANCE USE) HISTORY (page 6 of 13)
A. MIDDLE PERIOD (CONTINUED)

CLIENT'S FIRST NAME: Michelle   CLIENT'S ID NO. 92-SIL-01   DATE: 9-30-92

		None	1	2–5	6–10	10+
6.	**How many hospitalizations due to your use of:**					
	a. Alcohol	✓				
	b. Nicotine	✓				
	c. Caffeine	✓				
	d. Marijuana, euphoriants	✓				
	e. Stimulants, cocaine, amphetamines	✓				
	f. Depressants, tranquilizers, painkillers	✓				
	g. Hallucinogens, LSD, mushrooms, peyote, PCP	✓				
	h. Narcotics, barbiturates, other	✓				
7.	**How many arrests while driving have you had due to your use of:**					
	a. Alcohol	✓				
	b. Nicotine	✓				
	c. Caffeine	✓				
	d. Marijuana, euphoriants	✓				
	e. Stimulants, cocaine, amphetamines	✓				
	f. Depressants, tranquilizers, painkillers	✓				
	g. Hallucinogens, LSD, mushrooms, peyote, PCP	✓				
	h. Narcotics, barbiturates, other	✓				
8.	**How many times have you lost your driver's license due to the use of:**					
	a. Alcohol	✓				
	b. Nicotine	✓				
	c. Caffeine	✓				
	d. Marijuana, euphoriants	✓				
	e. Stimulants, cocaine, amphetamines	✓				
	f. Depressants, tranquilizers, painkillers	✓				
	g. Hallucinogens, LSD, mushrooms, peyote, PCP	✓				
	h. Narcotics, barbiturates, other	✓				
9.	**How many nondriving arrests due to the use of:**					
	a. Alcohol	✓				
	b. Nicotine	✓				
	c. Caffeine	✓				
	d. Marijuana, euphoriants	✓				
	e. Stimulants, cocaine, amphetamines	✓				
	f. Depressants, tranquilizers, painkillers	✓				
	g. Hallucinogens, LSD, mushrooms, peyote, PCP	✓				
	h. Narcotics, barbiturates, other	✓				

CONFIDENTIAL CHEMICAL (SUBSTANCE USE) HISTORY (page 7 of 13)
B. MIDDLE PERIOD (CONTINUED)

CLIENT'S FIRST NAME: Michelle	CLIENT'S ID NO. 92-51L-01		DATE: 9-30-92		
	None	1	2–5	6–10	10 +
10. How many arrests for violence due to the use of:					
a. Alcohol	✓				
b. Nicotine	✓				
c. Caffeine	✓				
d. Marijuana, euphoriants	✓				
e. Stimulants, cocaine, amphetamines	✓				
f. Depressants, tranquilizers, painkillers	✓				
g. Hallucinogens, LSD, mushrooms, peyote, PCP	✓				
h. Narcotics, barbiturates, other	✓				
11. How many ticket citations have you received while under the influence of:					
a. Alcohol		✓			
b. Nicotine	✓				
c. Caffeine	✓				
d. Marijuana, euphoriants	✓				
e. Stimulants, cocaine, amphetamines	✓				
f. Depressants, tranquilizers, painkillers	✓				
g. Hallucinogens, LSD, mushrooms, peyote, PCP	✓				
h. Narcotics, barbiturates, other	✓				
12. How many tickets have you received while NOT under the influence of:					
Alcohol, depressants, stimulants, marijuana, hallucinogens, or narcotics?	✓				
13. How many times have you been stopped by the police but not arrested while under the influence of:					
a. Alcohol	✓				
b. Nicotine	✓				
c. Caffeine	✓				
d. Marijuana, euphoriants	✓				
e. Stimulants, cocaine, amphetamines	✓				
f. Depressants, tranquilizers, painkillers	✓				
g. Hallucinogens, LSD, mushrooms, peyote, PCP	✓				
h. Narcotics, barbiturates, other	✓				

Form FPP-34-7/13-rev2/94 ©1994 GMS. Limited permission to photocopy only. For orders call (510) 865-5282, fax (510) 865-4295.

CONFIDENTIAL CHEMICAL (SUBSTANCE USE) HISTORY   (page 8 of 13)
B. MIDDLE PERIOD (CONTINUED)

CLIENT'S FIRST NAME: Michelle   CLIENT'S ID NO. 92-512-01   DATE: 9-30-92

		None	1	2–5	6–10	10 +
14.	**How many times did you miss work as a result of the use of:**					
	a. Alcohol		✓			
	b. Nicotine	✓				
	c. Caffeine	✓				
	d. Marijuana, euphoriants	✓				
	e. Stimulants, cocaine, amphetamines	✓				
	f. Depressants, tranquilizers, painkillers	✓				
	g. Hallucinogens, LSD, mushrooms, peyote, PCP	✓				
	h. Narcotics, barbiturates, other	✓				
15.	**How many times did you lose or change jobs as a result of the use of:**					
	a. Alcohol	✓				
	b. Nicotine	✓				
	c. Caffeine	✓				
	d. Marijuana, euphoriants	✓				
	e. Stimulants, cocaine, amphetamines	✓				
	f. Depressants, tranquilizers, painkillers	✓				
	g. Hallucinogens, LSD, mushrooms, peyote, PCP	✓				
	h. Narcotics, barbiturates, other	✓				
16.	**How many times have you been separated or divorced from a spouse or loved one due to the use of:**					
	a. Alcohol	✓				
	b. Nicotine	✓				
	c. Caffeine	✓				
	d. Marijuana, euphoriants	✓				
	e. Stimulants, cocaine, amphetamines	✓				
	f. Depressants, tranquilizers, painkillers	✓				
	g. Hallucinogens, LSD, mushrooms, peyote, PCP	✓				
	h. Narcotics, barbiturates, other	✓				

		Not at all	Mildly	Definitely	Extremely
17.	In your opinion, did your abuse of chemicals interfere with the style of life you wanted to lead?	✓			

CONFIDENTIAL CHEMICAL (SUBSTANCE USE) HISTORY (page 9 of 13)

CLIENT'S FIRST NAME: Michelle	CLIENT'S ID NO. 92-SIL-01	DATE: 9-30-92

Please answer the questions as they relate to the middle period of your substance use. Check all questions, even when substance use is similar in all periods. Please include nonprescription and prescription medications that affect your mood.

B. LATER PERIOD

		Never	1–4 times a year	5–12 times a year	2–7 times a month	2–4 times a week	5–7 times a week	Several times a day
1.	How many years does this period cover: 7							
2.	Your age at the start of this period: 28							
3.	How often did you use:							
	a. Alcohol				✓			
	b. Nicotine	✓						
	c. Caffeine						✓	
	d. Marijuana, euphoriants	✓						
	e. Stimulants, cocaine, amphetamines	✓						
	f. Depressants, tranquilizers, painkillers	✓						
	g. Hallucinogens, LSD, mushrooms, peyote, PCP	✓						
	h. Narcotics, barbiturates, other	✓						

4.	What was your maximum daily dose during your heaviest use of:	
	a. Alcohol 2 glasses of wine	b. Nicotine
	c. Caffeine 2 cups of coffee	d. Marijuana, euphoriants
	e. Stimulants, cocaine, amphetamines	f. Depressants, tranquilizers, painkillers
	g. Hallucinogens, etc.	h. Narcotics, barbiturates, other

5.	How many physical disabilities due to the use of:	None	One	2–5	6–10	10 +
	a. Alcohol	✓				
	b. Nicotine	✓				
	c. Caffeine	✓				
	d. Marijuana, euphoriants	✓				
	e. Stimulants, cocaine, amphetamines	✓				
	f. Depressants, tranquilizers, painkillers	✓				
	g. Hallucinogens, LSD, mushrooms, peyote, PCP	✓				
	h. Narcotics, barbiturates, other	✓				

CONFIDENTIAL CHEMICAL (SUBSTANCE USE) HISTORY   (page 10 of 13)
A. LATER PERIOD (CONTINUED)

CLIENT'S FIRST NAME: Michelle	CLIENT'S ID NO. 92-512-01		DATE: 9-30-92		

	None	1	2–5	6–10	10+
6. How many hospitalizations due to your use of:					
a. Alcohol	✓				
b. Nicotine	✓				
c. Caffeine	✓				
d. Marijuana, euphoriants	✓				
e. Stimulants, cocaine, amphetamines	✓				
f. Depressants, tranquilizers, painkillers	✓				
g. Hallucinogens, LSD, mushrooms, peyote, PCP	✓				
h. Narcotics, barbiturates, other	✓				
7. How many arrests while driving have you had due to your use of:					
a. Alcohol	✓				
b. Nicotine	✓				
c. Caffeine	✓				
d. Marijuana, euphoriants	✓				
e. Stimulants, cocaine, amphetamines	✓				
f. Depressants, tranquilizers, painkillers	✓				
g. Hallucinogens, LSD, mushrooms, peyote, PCP	✓				
h. Narcotics, barbiturates, other	✓				
8. How many times have you lost your driver's license due to the use of:					
a. Alcohol	✓				
b. Nicotine	✓				
c. Caffeine	✓				
d. Marijuana, euphoriants	✓				
e. Stimulants, cocaine, amphetamines	✓				
f. Depressants, tranquilizers, painkillers	✓				
g. Hallucinogens, LSD, mushrooms, peyote, PCP	✓				
h. Narcotics, barbiturates, other	✓				
9. How many nondriving arrests due to the use of:					
a. Alcohol	✓				
b. Nicotine	✓				
c. Caffeine	✓				
d. Marijuana, euphoriants	✓				
e. Stimulants, cocaine, amphetamines	✓				
f. Depressants, tranquilizers, painkillers	✓				
g. Hallucinogens, LSD, mushrooms, peyote, PCP	✓				
h. Narcotics, barbiturates, other	✓				

CONFIDENTIAL CHEMICAL (SUBSTANCE USE) HISTORY (page 11 of 13)
B. LATER PERIOD (CONTINUED)

CLIENT'S FIRST NAME: Michelle	CLIENT'S ID NO. 92-512-01	DATE: 9-30-92			
	None	1	2–5	6–10	10 +
10. How many arrests for violence due to the use of:					
a. Alcohol	✓				
b. Nicotine	✓				
c. Caffeine	✓				
d. Marijuana, euphoriants	✓				
e. Stimulants, cocaine, amphetamines	✓				
f. Depressants, tranquilizers, painkillers	✓				
g. Hallucinogens, LSD, mushrooms, peyote, PCP	✓				
h. Narcotics, barbiturates, other	✓				
11. How many ticket citations have you received while under the influence of:					
a. Alcohol	✓				
b. Nicotine	✓				
c. Caffeine	✓				
d. Marijuana, euphoriants	✓				
e. Stimulants, cocaine, amphetamines	✓				
f. Depressants, tranquilizers, painkillers	✓				
g. Hallucinogens, LSD, mushrooms, peyote, PCP	✓				
h. Narcotics, barbiturates, other	✓				
12. How many tickets have you received while NOT under the influence of:					
Alcohol, depressants, stimulants, marijuana, hallucinogens, or narcotics?			✓		
13. How many times have you been stopped by the police but not arrested while under the influence of:					
a. Alcohol	✓				
b. Nicotine	✓				
c. Caffeine	✓				
d. Marijuana, euphoriants	✓				
e. Stimulants, cocaine, amphetamines	✓				
f. Depressants, tranquilizers, painkillers	✓				
g. Hallucinogens, LSD, mushrooms, peyote, PCP	✓				
h. Narcotics, barbiturates, other	✓				

CONFIDENTIAL CHEMICAL (SUBSTANCE USE) HISTORY (page 12 of 13)
B. LATER PERIOD (CONTINUED)

CLIENT'S FIRST NAME: Michelle   CLIENT'S ID NO. 92-512-01   DATE: 9-30-92

	None	1	2–5	6–10	10 +
14. How many times did you miss work as a result of the use of:					
a. Alcohol	✓				
b. Nicotine	✓				
c. Caffeine	✓				
d. Marijuana, euphoriants	✓				
e. Stimulants, cocaine, amphetamines	✓				
f. Depressants, tranquilizers, painkillers	✓				
g. Hallucinogens, LSD, mushrooms, peyote, PCP	✓				
h. Narcotics, barbiturates, other	✓				
15. How many times did you lose or change jobs as a result of the use of:					
a. Alcohol	✓				
b. Nicotine	✓				
c. Caffeine	✓				
d. Marijuana, euphoriants	✓				
e. Stimulants, cocaine, amphetamines	✓				
f. Depressants, tranquilizers, painkillers	✓				
g. Hallucinogens, LSD, mushrooms, peyote, PCP	✓				
h. Narcotics, barbiturates, other	✓				
16. How many times have you been separated or divorced from a spouse or loved one due to the use of:					
a. Alcohol	✓				
b. Nicotine	✓				
c. Caffeine	✓				
d. Marijuana, euphoriants	✓				
e. Stimulants, cocaine, amphetamines	✓				
f. Depressants, tranquilizers, painkillers	✓				
g. Hallucinogens, LSD, mushrooms, peyote, PCP	✓				
h. Narcotics, barbiturates, other	✓				

	Not at all	Mildly	Definitely	Extremely
17. In your opinion, did your abuse of chemical interfere with the style of life you wanted to lead?	✓			

Form FPP-34-12/13-rev2/94 ©1994 GMS. Limited permission to photocopy only. For orders call (510) 865-5282, fax (510) 865-4295.

CONFIDENTIAL CHEMICAL (SUBSTANCE USE) HISTORY   (page 13 of 13)

CLIENT'S FIRST NAME: Michelle	CLIENT'S ID NO. 92-SIL-01	DATE: 9-30-92

D. SUBSTANCE USE HISTORY OF SIGNIFICANT OTHERS

		Never	1–2 times a year	5–12 times a year	2–7 times a month	2–4 times a week	5–7 times a week	Several times a day
1. Paternal Grandfather	Substance 1 Wine/Beer							✓
	Substance 2							
2. Paternal Grandmother	Substance 1 Wine						✓	
	Substance 2							
3. Maternal Grandfather	Substance 1 Liquor							
	Substance 2							
4. Maternal Grandmother	Substance 1	✓						
	Substance 2							
5. Father	Substance 1 Beer/Liquor						✓	
	Substance 2							
6. Mother	Substance 1 Wine/Beer						✓	
	Substance 2							
7. Brothers (5)	Substance 1 Wine/Liquor						✓	
	Substance 2							
8. Sisters (2)	Substance 1 Wine				✓			
	Substance 2							
9. Uncles	Substance 1 Wine/Beer						✓	
	Substance 2							
10. Aunts	Substance 1 Wine/Beer				✓			
	Substance 2							
11. Close Friends	Substance 1 Wine					✓		
	Substance 2 Cocaine				✓			
12. Your Spouse	Substance 1							
	Substance 2							
13. Your Children	Substance 1							
	Substance 2							

Form FPP-34-13/13-rev2/94 ©1994 GMS. Limited permission to photocopy only. For orders call (510) 865-5282, fax (510) 865-4295.

Confidential Sexual History
For evaluation of sexual functioning

As all clinicians know, sexual functioning can be clinically significant in determining diagnostic categories. This very thorough history is designed for both male and female clients and, depending on the transference, it may be more appropriately answered in a client's home rather than by direct interview. This form provides you with a most significant clinical choice: whether to have the client complete the form, or to fill it in yourself during direct interview. When using this form, consider transference issues and the focus, style, and techniques of the treatment.

The questions asked in the Confidential Sexual History are all in the form of check-off lists.

CONFIDENTIAL SEXUAL HISTORY · (page 1 of 5)

CLIENT'S FIRST NAME: Michelle	CLIENT'S ID NO. 92-SIL-01	DATE: 9-30-92

If you experience anxiety while attempting to answer any of the following questions, please circle the question.

	ANSWER ALL QUESTIONS AS BEST AS YOU CAN.	Never	Seldom	Occasionally	Frequently	Regularly
1.	Does the fact that you are male or female cause anxiety? (In other words, is your gender a source of discomfort?)	✓				
2.	Do you feel your sexual life is good and acceptable to you?		✓			
3.	Do you feel your sexual life is acceptable to the majority of society?				✓	
4.	Do you experience anxiety during sexual intercourse?			✓		
5.	Do you experience anxiety during sexual intercourse in your dreams or fantasies?	✓				
6.	Do you experience pain during sexual intercourse?	✓				
7.	Do you experience pain during sexual intercourse in your dreams or fantasies?	✓				
8.	Do you experience premature ejaculation during sexual intercourse?					
9.	Do you experience premature ejaculation during sexual intercourse in your dreams or fantasies?					
10.	Do you avoid getting sexually aroused?			✓		
11.	Do you avoid getting sexually aroused in your dreams or fantasies?	✓				
12.	Are you unable to get sexually aroused?			✓		
13.	Are you unable to get sexually aroused in your dreams or fantasies?	✓				
14.	If male, are you unable to get an erection?					

Form FPP-35-1/5-rev2/94 ©1994 GMS. Limited permission to photocopy only. For orders call (510) 865-5282, fax (510) 865-4295.

CONFIDENTIAL SEXUAL HISTORY   (page 2 of 5)

CLIENT'S FIRST NAME: Michelle	CLIENT'S ID NO. 92-51L-01		DATE: 9-30-92		

		Never	Seldom	Occasionally	Frequently	Regularly
15.	Are you unable to get an erection during your dreams or fantasies?					
16.	Do you experience orgasm?					✓
17.	Do you experience orgasm during your dreams or fantasies?					✓
18.	Do you experience orgasm, but not feel satisfied sexually?		✓			
19.	Do you experience orgasm, but not feel satisfied sexually in dreams or fantasies?	✓				
20.	Do you (or did you) experience premarital sexual intercourse?					✓
21.	Do you experience premarital sexual intercourse in dreams or fantasies?					✓
22.	If male, are you able to get an erection but not maintain to orgasm?					
23.	If male, are you able to get an erection but not maintain to orgasm in dreams or fantasies?					
24.	If male, are you unable to get an erection but able to experience orgasm?					
25.	If male, are you unable to get an erection but able to experience orgasm in dreams or fantasies?					
26.	Do you practice heterosexuality?					✓
27.	Do you practice heterosexuality in dreams or fantasies?					✓
28.	Do you practice homosexuality?	✓				
29.	Do you practice homosexuality in dreams or fantasies?	✓				
30.	Do you practice transvestism?	✓				
31.	Do you practice transvestism in dreams or fantasies?	✓				
32.	Do you practice bestiality (sex with animals)?	✓				
33.	Do you practice bestiality in dreams or fantasies?	✓				
34.	Do you practice oral sexual stimulation?			✓		

Form FPP-35-2/5-rev2/94 ©1994 GMS. Limited permission to photocopy only. For orders call (510) 865-5282, fax (510) 865-4295.

CONFIDENTIAL SEXUAL HISTORY   (page 3 of 5)

CLIENT'S FIRST NAME: Michelle	CLIENT'S ID NO. 92-S1L-01	DATE: 9-30-92

		Never	Seldom	Occasionally	Frequently	Regularly
35.	Do you practice oral sexual stimulation in dreams or fantasies?				✓	
36.	Do you practice anal intercourse?	✓				
37.	Do you practice anal intercourse in dreams or fantasies?	✓				
38.	Do you practice sadistic sex (inflicting pain)?	✓				
39.	Do you practice sadistic sex in dreams or fantasies?	✓				
40.	Do you practice masochistic sex (receiving pain)?	✓				
41.	Do you practice masochistic sex in dreams or fantasies?	✓				
42.	Do you practice voyeurism (watching others to get sexually aroused)?			✓		
43.	Do you practice voyeurism in dreams or fantasies?			✓		
44.	Do you practice peeking, as in "Peeping Tom"?	✓				
45.	Do you practice peeking in dreams or fantasies?			✓		
46.	Do you practice incest (sex with close relatives)?	✓				
47.	Do you practice incest in dreams or fantasies?	✓				
48.	Do you have sexual interest in children?	✓				
49.	Do you have sexual interest in children in dreams or fantasies?	✓				
50.	Do you have sexual interest primarily in people younger than you?				✓	
51.	Do you have sexual interest primarily in people younger than you in dreams or fantasies?					✓
52.	Do you have sexual interest primarily in people older than you?		✓			
53.	Do you have sexual interest primarily in people older than you in dreams or fantasies?		✓			
54.	Do you have sexual interest primarily in objects rather than persons?	✓				

Form FPP-35-3/5-rev2/94 ©1994 GMS. Limited permission to photocopy only. For orders call (510) 865-5282, fax (510) 865-4295.

CONFIDENTIAL SEXUAL HISTORY   (page 4 of 5)

CLIENT'S FIRST NAME: Michelle	CLIENT'S ID NO. 92-51L-01	DATE: 9-30-92

		Never	Seldom	Occasionally	Frequently	Regularly
55.	Do you have a sexual interest primarily in objects rather than persons in dreams or fantasies?	✓				
56.	Have any other than the above been part of your sex experience? (List and give frequency for each)					
57.	Have any of the practices listed in 56 been part of your sex experience in dreams or fantasies? (List for each)					
58.	Have you had sexual experiences during blackouts (loss of memory)?	✓				

		Never	Seldom	Occasionally	Frequently	Regularly	Cause Anxiety? Yes	No
59.	Do you presently practice sexual intercourse with your spouse or lover:		✓				✓	
60.	Do you presently practice sexual intercourse with your spouse or lover in dreams or fantasies:		✓					✓
61.	Do you practice sexual intercourse with anyone other than your spouse or lover?	✓						✓
62.	Do you practice sexual intercourse with anyone other than your spouse or lover in dreams or fantasies?		✓				✓	
63.	Do you consider your sexual practices promiscuous?	✓						✓
64.	Have you practiced masturbation in the past?				✓			✓
65.	Do you practice masturbation presently?				✓			✓
66.	If female, do you fear pregnancy?				✓		✓	
67.	If male, do you fear impregnating your sexual partner?							
68.	Do you use contraception?				✓		✓	

CONFIDENTIAL SEXUAL HISTORY   (page 5 of 5)

CLIENT'S FIRST NAME: Michelle	CLIENT'S ID NO. 92-SIL-01	DATE: 9-30-92

69.	What was your age when you first experienced sexual intercourse? 18
70.	If female, how many pregnancies have you had? 2
71.	If female, how many births? None
72.	How many children were you responsible for raising? None
73.	How many abortions by choice have you experienced? 2
74.	How many abortions NOT by choice have you experienced?

		None	Mild	Definite	Extreme
75.	Anxiety as a result of abortions by choice:			✓	
76.	Anxiety as a result of abortions NOT by choice:				
77.	Have you experienced anxiety about contracting a veneral disease?	✓			
78.	Have you experienced anxiety about contracting AIDS?		✓		

		Never	Once	2–5 times	5–10 times	10–20 times	Over 20
79.	How many times have you had gonorrhea?	✓					
80.	How often have you had syphilis?	✓					

81.	If female, what was your age at onset of menstruation? 11 Years
82.	Character of your menses? (Regular) Irregular
83.	Amount of flow: Minimal (Moderate) Excessive

		Never	Seldom	Occasionally	Frequently	Regularly
84.	If female, do you experience discomfort during menses?			✓		
85.	For both male and female, do you practice intercourse during menses?	✓				
86.	Does practicing intercourse during menses cause discomfort or anxiety?					✓
87.	Do you experience anxiety because you feel your sexual organs are undersized?	✓				
88.	Do you experience anxiety because you feel your sexual organs are oversized?	✓				
89.	Do you experience anxiety because you feel you are undersexed?			✓		
90.	Do you experience anxiety because you feel you are oversexed?	✓				
91.	Do you ever experience anxiety about being born the wrong gender?	✓				

Form FPP35-5/5-rev2/94 ©1994 GMS. Limited permission to photocopy only. For orders call (510) 865-5282, fax (510) 865-4295.

6

Writing Your Reports
Samples of Written Reports

In this chapter we examine three separate reports written by three different professionals working on the same case. Each report begins with an overview of the format to be used and then includes a sample of the completed report. These are formats used by medical and nonmedical health practitioners. They meet the report-writing criteria of the American Psychological Association for insurance companies, civil suits, and the State of California Workers' Compensation Board.

No matter what format you choose as necessary for your client's protection, I cannot emphasize enough the importance of working with a team of other experts when preparing a case for hearing. Over the years, I have stressed to university students, interns, and anyone who will listen: I don't treat a client. *We* treat a client.

One of the fundamental responsibilities of a private practice clinician is to develop professional resources in many areas of expertise so that you can ensure that clients receive the best of care and the care they need. When preparing for a legal case, you will find it necessary to work with testing psychologists, physicians, and psychiatrists. You will also (with your client's permission) want to consult with your client's attorney so that you can accurately report your clinical findings in a forensic setting. For example, in most forensic settings the hearing officers and judge will rely heavily on the summation or recommendation section of your report. By conferring with your client's attorney you can find out what specific summation points and recommendations, based on your clinical findings, will serve your client best. You can then incorporate these as appropriate into your report summation.

I remember one case in which the attorney asked if I could estimate my client's future need for psychotherapy and the cost of that therapy and rehabilitation. If I had not asked my client's attorney for input, I would never have thought to add such estimates to my summation—even though I had recommended further psychotherapy and rehabilitation. Researching the costs helped my client's attorney secure an award for my client that enabled her to recover from both the physical and emotional injuries she had suffered.

When an insurance company asks me to prepare a report to aid them in determining the continuance of payments for psychotherapeutic services (by peer or utilization review), I have found that by speaking to the professionals working for the insurance company in their review section, I am able to focus on the clinical information they need. In general, I have found that private practitioners, as well as personnel working in institutions, are highly cooperative in helping structure clinical arguments. In this rather lonely profession, where typically we are working with an individual client or family, we need all the help we can get.

Finally, I pose to you a question asked of me over 25 years ago by a supervisor of my clinical training: "Michael," he said, "are you taking as good care of yourself as you are of your clients?" One way of taking care of yourself is to take care of your clients by using collegial support systems.

Are you taking as good care of yourself as you are of your clients?

Mental Health Treatment Report

This report illustrates how to respond to insurance inquiries and legal inquiries. The example situation revolves around a worker's compensation hearing and a concomitant lawsuit that a mythical Michelle Silver files against her employer. George R. Jones, Ph.D., is Ms. Silver's treating psychotherapist, and he writes the following treatment report.

The report consists of the following items:

Item 1.   Letter acknowledging request for report

Item 2.   Itemized billing statement

Item 3.   Billing statement

Item 4.   Mental Health Treatment Report; which includes the following sections:

1. Diagnosis (DSM III-R)
2. Client's Initial Reason for Seeking Treatment
3. Work History (not required for non–work-related reports)
4. Mental Status Examination
5. Course of Treatment
6. Collateral Contacts
7. Current Treatment Goals
8. Summation, Prognosis, and Recommendations

GEORGE R. JONES, Ph.D.
1234 W. Main Blvd., Suite 5
Los Angeles CA 90000
(213) 555-1212 (213) 555-1213

SAMPLE

August 26, 1993

David Stein
A Law Corporation
4625 Park Avenue
Los Angeles CA 91234

Dear Mr. Stein:

I am in receipt of your request for a complete Mental Health Treatment Report regarding your client, Michelle Silver. I am also in receipt of Ms. Silver's release of information.

Enclosed is an itemized statement for services rendered, a photocopy of my original clinical notes, and a billing statement for this report. If I may be of further assistance to you in this matter, please call.

I remain respectfully yours,

George R. Jones, Ph.D.
M.V. 4011

Enclosure

GRJ/ll

SAMPLE

GEORGE R. JONES, PH.D.
1234 Main Blvd., Suite 5
Los Angeles, California 90000
(213) 555-1212 (310) 555-1213

ITEMIZED BILLING STATEMENT

Re: Michelle Silver
1992–93

All billing (unless otherwise noted) is for one, 50-minute psychotherapy session (RVS 90803) at my rate of $90.00 per session. (Since Ms. Silver is currently in treatment, this does not represent a final statement of billing.)

1992

August	25	90.00
September	15, 26, 30	270.00
October	2, 9, 16	270.00
November	6, 13, 20	270.00
December	4, 11, 18	270.00

December 18 brief report for
National Insurance Company 160.00

Total 1992 = $1,330.00

1993

January	23, 30	180.00
February	5, 12, 19, 26	360.00
March	5, 12, 19, 26	360.00
April	2, 9, 23, 30	360.00
May	7, 21, 28	270.00
June	4, 18	180.00
July	9, 16, 23, 30	360.00
August	20	90.00

September 26 report for Attorney 525.00

Total 1993 = $2,685.00

TOTAL BILLING AS OF 9/26/93 = $4,015.00

GEORGE R. JONES, Pd.D.
1234 W. Main Blvd., Suite 5
Los Angeles, CA 90000
(213) 555-1212 (213) 555-1213

BILLING STATEMENT

Service: Mental Health Treatment Report
For client: Michelle Silver
Requested by: David Stein
Report dated: 9/26/93

Service rendered included:

    review of records
    photocopying of appropriate materials
    steno and typing services
    report writing

Total billing = $525.00

Please remit directly to my office at the above address.

Mental Health Treatment Report

George R. Jones, Ph.D.
September 27, 1993

MICHELLE SILVER

1. DIAGNOSIS (DSM-III-R)

Axis I:	307.42	Insomnia Disorder (related to another mental disorder—nonorganic)
	296.33	Major Depression—recurrent and severe without psychotic features
Axis II:	799.90	Diagnosis deferred
Axis III:		See medical and psychiatric reports
Axis IV:	4	Severity of psychosocial stressor scale: adult
Axis V:	Current GAF:	40 Global assessment of functioning scale. Some impairment in reality testing and communication, and major impairment in several areas including work, family relations, judgment, thinking, and mood.
	Highest GAF past year:	50–60 Moderate to serious symptoms including difficulty in family relationships and social and occupational functioning, as well as labile affect and suicidal ideation.

2. CLIENT'S INITIAL REASON FOR SEEKING TREATMENT

Ms. Silver, a former client, reported for psychotherapy on September 26, 1992. She stated that she felt depressed because she might have serious damage to her body as a result of an auto accident she was involved in on August 26, 1992. The client clearly presented a complete clinical picture of moderate to severe depression and was referred to a psychiatrist, Robert Young, M.D., for medical evaluation.

The client reported that the accident occurred while she was making a delivery to the bank for her employer, when she was struck on the driver's side of her car. The client said she had obtained medical treatment following the accident. Client was concerned that she couldn't go back to work. Client presented a clinical picture of confusion and emotional lability. The client later stated during therapy that as a result of the accident, her employer accused her of "acting peculiar" and fired her.

Mental Health Treatment Report
Michelle Silver
9/26/93
Page 2 of 4

3. WORK HISTORY (not required for non–work-related reports)

Client presents a picture of working since she was 15 years of age when she began working in a laundry. Her early education took place in Oregon. After coming to California with her family, she studied nursing at St. Mary's Hospital in Torrance, California. She worked as a nurse's aide for nine years. It was at this time that client sought vocational counseling from me. She was looking for a career in which she wouldn't have to spend so much time on her feet. As a result of the counseling, she took courses in bookkeeping and accounting (for one year) and then worked for A.D.S. Inc., a property management firm, for two and a half years. She then worked at an electronics company, and was subsequently employed by E & M Computers, Inc., earning $1,600 per month. Client returned to therapy after the accident, this time requiring psychotherapy for her depression.

4. MENTAL STATUS EXAMINATION

Ms. Silver is a 35-year-old Caucasian female. Her date of birth is September 21, 1958. She was born in Oregon. She is 5'8" tall and her current weight is 170 lbs.

During the course of treatment, which began on September 26, 1992, her weight has fluctuated downward. The client appears older or younger than her actual age, reflecting her fluctuations in weight. Her appearance is tall with a medium to heavy build, and her pupils are equal. Her hygienic state is clean and her clothing is neat. Her posture fluctuates from normal to slumped, and her facial expressions vary from tense to sad to worried. Her attitude and behavior vary from alert to confused. Her attention span is poor to satisfactory. Eye contact is avoidant. Muscular movements are hypoactive. There are no unusual mannerisms. She frequently cries, although her demeanor fluctuates from friendly and trustful to evasive. She is reserved and basically cooperative. Her mood is anxious, fearful, suspicious, depressed, and angry. Her affect is labile but generally appropriate to content.

Client's mother tongue is English and she understands Spanish. The quality of her speech is normal to slow. There are no impediments. The content varies from concrete to circumstantial. Her thought and associations vary from logical to blocking. Her appetite is poor.

During the course of therapy, there was significant weight loss and her sleep was characterized by early-morning wakefulness. Client reports no drug use.

Her judgment fluctuates from poor to adequate. Her estimated intelligence is above average. Her thought content is sometimes persecutory. There are no hallucinations, no

Mental Health Treatment Report
Michelle Silver
9/26/93
Page 3 of 4

SAMPLE

illusions, and no ideas of reference. There is some perseveration and some obsessive/compulsive behavior in regard to cleanliness. Suicidal ideation was present at time of initial interview and had recurred occasionally throughout the course of therapy. While motivation for treatment is high, her insight is poor. Client is oriented to time, place, and person. There is some memory impairment. Her general knowledge is adequate.

5. COURSE OF TREATMENT

The course of treatment for this client varied. For the most part the client reported on a once-a-week basis and was cooperative and compliant during interviews. She was apparently taking the medications prescribed by Dr. Young, and there was a definite improvement in attitude and affect.

Beginning in late July to early August of 1993, the client relapsed into a major depression. Upon consultation, her medications were reviewed and changed. This relapse may have been an anniversary response to her auto accident and subsequent firing. The client missed several sessions between 7/30/93 and 8/18/93 and came late to several sessions thereafter. The client made several phone calls after 11 p.m. indicating feelings of panic. During the course of treatment, I have kept closely in touch with Dr. Young informing him of client's lability. As of our last session held 9/20/93, the client seems to be a little improved, but my prognosis is guarded.

6. COLLATERAL CONTACTS

Robert Young, M.D.
2201 Center Boulevard
Los Angeles, CA 90000
(213) 444-3333

7. CURRENT TREATMENT GOALS

1. Stabilize affect.
2. Ameliorate depressive symptomatology.
3. Enhance compliance with medical regimens.
4. Futurize a plan to expand social and work networks and support systems.
5. Reestablish self-esteem in relation to work environment.
6. Reestablish sense of trust in work and social environments.

8. SUMMATION, PROGNOSIS, AND RECOMMENDATIONS

My prognosis for this client's recovery at this time is guarded. Her recovery will depend on several factors: her ability to comply with medical regimens and psychotherapy; her ability to regain a sense of self-esteem and trust in relation to the work environment; her gaining support from family and social networking, as well as from the various institutions and agencies that can provide economic and rehabilitative support. This client may need to remain on medications (based on my consultation with Dr. Young) for an extended period of time (one year plus). Psychotherapy will need to be continued on a once- to twice-a-week basis for a minimum of two years. Vocational rehabilitation and retraining may be required. If all of the above factors can be attended to and provided for this client, my prognosis would change to good.

This client presents a similar clinical picture to that of a posttraumatic stress disorder client, usually seen as a result of having participated in a catastrophic event such as war. Sensitive handling of all aspects of this case, i.e., medical, psychological, and vocational rehabilitation, is definitely required to ensure recovery.

Psychological Report

This sample report is prepared by a clinical psychologist, Dr. Cynthia Roberts, who specializes in testing and report writing related to disability findings. Because of Dr. Roberts' expertise in this area and her experience with consulting for hearings and other forensic situations, Dr. Jones refers his client to her for testing.

You may find the format used in this report helpful in formulating your reports. I recommend that you write your report out of sequence. Write those sections that are easiest first. Write the summation after all the material is presented.

The psychological report format used by Dr. Roberts contains the following sections:

1. Psychodiagnostic Evaluation

2. Pertinent History

3. Review of Medical Records

4. Behavioral Observations

5. Tests Administered

6. Test Results and Interpretation

7. Intellectual Functioning

8. Emotional Functioning

9. Results and Discussion

10. Diagnostic Impressions

11. Recommendations

Psychological Report

SAMPLE

PAIGE PSYCHOLOGICAL SERVICES
8765 West Street
Los Angeles, CA 91234

March 14, 1994

Mr. David Stein
Attorney at Law
4625 Park Avenue
Los Angeles, CA 91234

> EMP: E & M Computers, Inc.
> WCAB: 93 ABC 1234
> D/I: C.T. 10/91–10/92

PSYCHODIAGNOSTIC EVALUATION

Dear Mr. Stein:

I have completed the psychological evaluation at the request of Dr. Robert Young to help in the assessment of Ms. Silver's current emotional status. This procedure included a clinical interview with the client as well as a battery of objective and projective tests that were administered to Ms. Silver on March 9, 1994. The entire testing session took approximately four-and-a-half hours.

PERTINENT HISTORY

Ms. Silver is a 35-year-old woman who was born in Oregon and lived there until the age of 15. In 1974 she moved to California with her family.

Ms. Silver is the second youngest of eight children. She has two sisters and five brothers. One of her brothers died in an automobile accident in 1988. Both her parents are alive and well; her father is 75 and her mother is 65.

Ms. Silver states that her father came from Italy where he worked for the military for 17 years and then as a driver for the transit system.

Ms. Silver attended high school in Los Angeles. From 1976 to 1985 Ms. Silver worked at St. Mary's Hospital, first in the kitchen and then as a practical nurse. She states that she received her training as a nurse's aide at St. Mary's Hospital in Torrance. She claims to have enjoyed her work and was very sensitive to the clients' needs.

In 1985 Ms. Silver went back to school, at a business college, and trained in bookkeeping and accounting. She was then placed in a property management firm, working for A.D.S., Inc., for two-and-a-half years, doing accounting.

Ms. Silver reports that in 1990 she got another job at an electronics company. She worked there until the management went out of business.

Psychological Report
Michelle Silver
3/14/94
Page 2 of 11

From January of 1991 to October of 1992 the client worked for E & M Computers, Inc. as a bookkeeper. Ms. Silver reports that initially she liked her job. At first they were situated in Los Angeles in an old building that was "falling apart." Evidently, they moved to another setting on Santa Monica Boulevard, and she was quite instrumental in setting the place up for business. Unfortunately, her boss was evicted for not paying his rent. Finally, they moved to one small room that housed six employees. Ms. Silver claims that in spite of all these changes, she made an effort to remain organized and consistent. However, what bothered her the most was her boss's attitude and lack of consideration. Ms. Silver claims that he frequently yelled at her, particularly when he failed to "take care of his own business." In addition, she was frequently yelled at by customers who did not get paid for their services.

As a result of cumulative work-related stress, the client sought treatment with Dr. George Jones, for short-term supportive psychotherapy. In May of 1992 she was also referred to Dr. Young to be evaluated for antidepressants.

Ms. Silver claims that the pressure kept mounting and finally, on August 26, 1992, her boss sent her with a check to pay for an overdue mortgage payment on his condo. On the way back to work, the client was involved in a car accident. She claims to have hit her head against the side door. A week later she returned to work, but was experiencing severe symptoms of anxiety, depression, headaches, and nightmares about the accident, and she could not maintain long working hours. Furthermore, the client claimed that at that point she did not care much about herself or her work. In October of 1992, she was fired from her job. She has not worked since that time.

Ms. Silver is a single woman. At the present time she is living with her nephew (the son of her deceased brother). For a time she lived with a boyfriend; that relationship ended in the winter of 1992. She claims that although the relationship had its own drawbacks, her work-related difficulties were a contributing factor to its downfall.

At the present time the client spends most of her time at home. She claims that she does not sleep well at night, being awakened frequently by nightmares. Her mood fluctuates a great deal. She is often irritable, angry, lethargic, has difficulty concentrating on details, and finds herself crying about minor issues. She reports that since the car accident she has been experiencing numbness in some areas of her legs. She claims that the neurologist diagnosed her symptoms as a pinched nerve.

For the past year and a half, the client has been under psychiatric treatment, both for medication and psychotherapy. She sees Dr. George Jones for ongoing supportive psycho-therapy on a once-a-week basis. She sees Dr. Robert Young for pharmacological management.

The client's medical history includes gall bladder surgery at the age of 22, surgery on her feet at the age of 25, and two abortions, the last one taking place when she was 30 years old. The client reports that she does not use recreational drugs, does not smoke, and occasionally drinks during social gatherings.

Psychological Report
Michelle Silver
3/14/94
Page 3 of 11

REVIEW OF MEDICAL RECORDS

Following the August 1992 car accident, the client was referred to Dr. Irene Phillips, a neurologist, for an evaluation. In her September 30, 1992 report, she diagnosed the client as having had:

1. Postconcussion headache, acute
2. Tension-muscle contraction headache
3. Blepharospasm
4. Meralgia Paresthetica
5. Tinnitus

In Dr. Young's report of January 21, 1994, he diagnosed the client as having major depression, single episode and posttraumatic stress disorder.

Dr. Robert Thomas, a psychiatrist, evaluated the client on December 7, 1993 for the Department of Social Services. He diagnosed the client as having "dysthymic disorder, moderately severe, accompanied by a great deal of anxiety, tension, frustration, insomnia . . . this client's main limitation seems to be that she's attempting to deal with her anger and irritation through the mechanism of depression."

BEHAVIORAL OBSERVATIONS

Ms. Silver arrived early for her appointment. She looked her stated age and was neatly dressed and groomed. She was oriented to all spheres and evidenced no observable signs of gross physical motor impairment or florid thought disorder. During the early phase of the evaluation, the client appeared to be somewhat apprehensive about the testing process. However, she gradually began to feel more comfortable with me, and became more friendly and revealing about herself. She admitted that she did not sleep well the night before, and that she was worried about her performance during the evaluation today.

Ms. Silver made the effort to cooperate thoroughly with the various tasks. Whenever she recognized that her performance was less than adequate, she became quite frustrated and embarrassed. While giving history, she frequently ran into difficulties in providing a proper sequence of events. During the course of the evaluation, there were observable signs of anxiety, disappointment, and feelings of inadequacy.

At the end of the testing process, the client shared with me her predicament and concern about her future. She claims that at the present time she sees herself as being more depressed than at any other time in her life. She admits that she had experienced some form of depression in her past, but in the last couple of years the depression seems to have "totally taken over." Currently she finds herself wanting to be left alone, and not to get involved socially. Furthermore, she claims that her concentration has become extremely poor. She frequently finds herself getting irritable, short-tempered, anxious, and experiencing headaches, stomach trouble, and leg pain.

Psychological Report
Michelle Silver
3/14/94
Page 4 of 11

Ms. Silver recognizes that she has benefited a great deal from the psychiatric treatment and that she will need to remain under medical attention for a while to come. Furthermore, she expresses interest in vocational rehabilitation. She claims that she does not want to go back to accounting and that she would like to get training in an area such as travel management. Ms. Silver states that she recognizes the need to get out of "this rut I'm in." She admits to having suicidal ideations, without the intent to carry. She claims that even during the testing she was "tuning out": "sometimes I don't hear what people tell me, my concentration and memory is not good anymore."

TESTS ADMINISTERED

Wechsler Adult Intelligence Scale—Revised (WAIS-R)

Wechsler Memory Scale, Form 1

Rorschach Ink Blot Test

Thematic Apperception Test (TAT)

Minnesota Multiphasic Personality Inventory (MMPI)

(Will compare her current MMPI results with those obtained from her at this office on October 22, 1993.)

TEST RESULTS AND INTERPRETATION

Wechsler Adult Intelligence Scale—Revised (WAIS-R)

Verbal Subtests	Scaled Scores
Information	10
Digit Span	8
Vocabulary	11
Arithmetic	7
Comprehension	16
Similarities	13

Performance Subtests	Scaled Scores
Picture Completion	9
Picture Arrangement	6
Block Design	8
Object Assembly	7
Digit Symbol	8
Verbal	105
Performance	89
Full Scale IQ	98

INTELLECTUAL FUNCTIONING

The Wechsler scores are standardized so that the average person scores consistently across the subtests, with the mid-average score being 10. Some variation is normal. However, when it exceeds a certain level, we infer an acquired intellectual impairment, in which high subtest scores reflect premorbid intelligence and low scores reflect the areas affected by psychological or organic disturbances.

On the WAIS-R, Ms. Silver obtained scores that placed her in the average range of intelligence. Her full-scale score was 98, with a verbal score of 105 and a performance score of 89. This places her in the fiftieth percentile of the population with regard to current intellectual functioning. Her data indicate that she shows more strength in the verbal section of the test, verbal score being 16 points above her performance score. This difference is statistically significant. A discrepancy of this magnitude, particularly since the verbal is higher than the performance, is most likely related to emotional symptoms such as anxiety and depression, which are known to lower scores. To support this evidence, her lower scores were in the areas that rely heavily on concentration and speed.

A verbal score higher than a performance score could also be associated with right-hemisphere impairment or brain damage. I would like to bring this up, particularly in the light that this client did experience a head concussion during the August 1992 car accident. However, I would like to emphasize that because she consistently scored low on the performance subtests, her results are more likely to be related to psychological factors such as anxiety and depression rather than to brain damage.

Ms. Silver's highest scores among the 11 subtests that also fell well above the average range are in the following areas:

1. Comprehension: This requires the subject to use conventional wisdom and judgment. Her very high score of 16 in this area reveals that she is capable of using common sense and applying past experiences to present situations.

2. Similarities: Her high score of 13 here suggests that she is capable of logical and abstract thinking.

3. Vocabulary: Vocabulary is considered one of the most stable aspects of intelligence and thus is one of the last subtests to be affected by emotional disturbances or brain damage. Her score of 11 here indicates that her intellectual endowment is above average.

The scores that fell far below Ms. Silver's own average were in the following areas:

1. Object Assembly: This subtest is a measure of visual, spatial organizational ability, reflecting the speed component as well. Here, the client obtained a score of 7, one of her lowest among the 11 subtests.

Psychological Report
Michelle Silver
3/14/94
Page 6 of 11

2. Digit Symbol: Digit Symbol measures speed, accuracy, and immediate memory. A low score can be associated with conditions ranging from anxiety to brain damage. Here, Ms. Silver earned a score of 8, one of her lowest among the 11 subtests.

3. Arithmetic: This subtest measures concentration, attention, and problem-solving skills. Here, Ms. Silver earned a score of 7, again, one of her lowest scores. This particular subtest is also known to vary considerably with anxiety and depression.

4. Picture Arrangement: This subtest measures visual perception and planning ability. The client's very low score of 6 indicates weakness in this area.

5. Block Design: This requires a subject to reproduce design from pattern-visual perception. This particular subtest is known to vary with organicity or emotional difficulties. Her low score of 8 on this subtest again suggests a weakness in this area.

Ms. Silver was also given the Wechsler Memory Scale. Here, the client obtained a MQ (Mental Quotient) of 120, which in all probability is a better representative of this client's premorbid intellectual endowment than her score on the WAIS-R. Her overall scores on the various tasks fell above the average range. However, Ms. Silver did rather poorly with the Digit Span subtest of the Wechsler Memory Scale.

On both the Wechsler Memory Scale and the WAIS-R Intelligence Scale, the client obtained poor scores on digit backward. The digit backward test requires the brief storing of few data bits while juggling them around mentally. This is an effortful activity that calls upon the working memory, as distinct from the more passive span of apprehension, measured by digit forward. Organically related difficulties, or emotional problems such as anxiety and depression, tend to reduce the number of digits recalled.

In summary, at the present time, Ms. Silver appears to be functioning at the average range of intelligence. However, her high scores on the verbal portion of the WAIS-R clearly suggest that in all probability, prior to the recent car accident and work-related difficulties, the client had functioned at a higher cognitive level, at least at the high average range of intelligence. However, she is now functioning at a lower cognitive level, and in all probability it is related to the emotional symptoms that she is currently manifesting; namely, anxiety and depression, which are known to lower many of the scores. At the present time the client shows definite weaknesses in areas that relate to visual spatial ability, immediate memory, speed, and concentration.

EMOTIONAL FUNCTIONING

Projective Testing

The results obtained from the projective testing, the Rorschach and Thematic Apperception Test (TAT), indicate that this individual has an intact ego in good contact with reality. Furthermore, they reveal that her quality of thinking is generally orderly, creative, and

Psychological Report
Michelle Silver
3/14/94
Page 7 of 11

realistic. When asked to tell stories to TAT cards, her responses show the abilities to perceive conventional aspects of her world and to organize her stories in a meaningful way that include a beginning, middle, and end.

Typically, the projective stimuli attempt to elicit information as to how an individual perceives his or her environment. The major theme that permeated the projective evaluation was generally one of sadness, loneliness, and the fear of illness or death.

On the TAT cards, the client saw people crying, angry, hiding their feelings, and receiving bad news. For example, on one of the TAT cards she saw a young boy playing a violin: "He looks sad, he is not concentrating, and he is preoccupied." On another TAT card she saw a young girl who "is not paying attention, her mind is somewhere else, she is tired." On another card she saw a detective telling an elderly woman "bad news."

On the Rorschach protocol the client made the attempt to distance herself from situations, yet her responses revealed the need for closeness and affection.

The client's responses to both the TAT and the Rorschach protocol indicated that she is capable of entering into interpersonal relationships and that she has the capacity to show remorse and genuine feelings in regard to familial obligations. Furthermore, her responses suggest that she is making an effort to look at the positive side of things.

In summary, Ms. Silver's overall projective responses reveal that she has an intact ego in good contact with reality. Her quality of thinking is generally orderly and creative. They further suggest that at the present time her tolerance of stress is limited, yet she is aware of her limitations and the need to change things. There is no bizarreness to indicate the presence of thought disorder or sociopathic tendency. However, the client does show elements of anxiety, worry, suspiciousness, morbid themes, and concern in regard to her future.

Personality Profile

Validity Scales:	L	F	K							
Current T Scores:	45	78	40							
10/22/93 Results:	53	83	42							
Clinical Scales:	Hs	D	Hy	Pd	Mf	Pa	Pt	Sc	Ma	Si
Current T Scores:	70	85	64	95	52	87	87	85	70	75
10/22/93 Results:	82	85	68	93	52	100	72	80	87	68

Ms. Silver was given the MMPI on two separate occasions. The first was in October of 1993, and the second was during this current evaluation. On both occasions the client obtained a valid profile. What this means is that she made an attempt to read the instructions carefully, and that her responses appear to be realistic and truthful and are likely to reflect her current status. In a nonclient population, the norm for the clinical scales tends to fall between 45 and 60. The results from the client's October 1993 MMPI indicate the following:

Psychological Report
Michelle Silver
3/14/94
Page 8 of 11

SAMPLE

At that time, the client was highly suspicious, agitated, anxious, significantly depressed, and intensely worried about her health. Also, she was undergoing some cognitive disorganization and experiencing mood fluctuation. The breakdown of the various clinical scales are provided above.

On her current MMPI, the client also obtained high elevations. The scores that fell well above the normal range on the current administration are as follows:

1. Physical Worries and Complaints (Scale Hs, 1): Her score of 70 here suggests that at the present time she is intensely worried about her health. On the MMPI she notes that she feels weak all over, experiences stomach trouble and headaches, and is unable to work.

2. Level of Depression (Scale D, 2): Her score of 85 here suggests that at the present time she is significantly depressed. On the MMPI she identifies that she cries easily, sometimes feels as if she must injure herself, feels useless, and has trouble with memory and concentration.

3. Conformity to Moral Standards (Scale Pd, 4): Her score of 95 here suggests that she may be experiencing some difficulty with a figure in authority.

4. Level of Suspiciousness and Paranoia (Scale Pa, 6): Her score of 87 here suggests that at the present time she is highly suspicious and sensitive to criticism. On the MMPI she notes that someone has it in for her and that she is being plotted against.

5. Level of Anxiety and Ruminative Worries (Scale Pt, 7): Her score of 87 here suggests that at the present time she is worried, tense, and indecisive. On the MMPI she identifies that she feels anxious about something or someone almost all of the time.

6. Level of Mental Confusion (Scale Sc, 8): Her score of 85 here suggests that at the present time she may have feelings of isolation and problems with logic and concentration. Furthermore, her Jonesberg Index of 66 places the profile in the psychotic direction. This does not necessary mean that this client is psychotic, but because of her distress, her perception of reality is rather tenuous. In fact, on the MMPI she continued to admit that something is wrong with her mind and that she is afraid of losing it.

7. Level of Mood Fluctuation (Scale Ma, 9): Her score of 70 here suggests that she is highly agitated and may go through extended periods of sleep disturbances.

The MMPI literature suggests that clients who generate this type of profile present symptoms of depression, anxiousness, worriedness, multiple fears, apprehensiveness, blunting of expression or affect, concreteness of thinking, and morbid rumination. There is also a tendency toward an extreme sensitivity to criticisms. These types of clients tend to have suicidal ideations and present a high level of physical symptoms. A common diagnosis for such a client is one of depression. Psychotherapy tends to be slow but can help her work through her unrealistically high self-expectations and her inability to express anger out of fear or guilt.

Psychological Report
Michelle Silver
3/14/94
Page 9 of 11

In summary, Ms. Silver was administered two MMPIs, five months apart. Her profiles reveal similar findings. Although the client appears to be somewhat less suspicious than she did five months ago, her overall symptoms continue to present a picture of an individual who is significantly depressed, highly suspicious, and intensely worried about her health. Also, she is experiencing a high level of agitation, anxiety, and cognitive disorganization.

RESULTS AND DISCUSSION

Ms. Michelle Silver is a 35-year-old woman who was born and raised in Oregon. She completed her high school education in Los Angeles and worked for a number of years at St. Mary's Hospital in the capacity of nurse's aide. She then furthered her education and got training in bookkeeping and accounting.

From January of 1991 to October of 1992, Ms. Silver worked for E & M Computers, Inc. as a bookkeeper. She reports that in spite of the frequent moves the company made, she made the effort to be consistent and reliable. However, work-related problems eventually escalated. Her boss would frequently misdirect his anger at her and she was yelled at by her boss and by contractors who did not get paid for their services.

As a result of cumulative work-related stress, the client sought treatment with Dr. George Jones for supportive psychotherapy. In May of 1992, she was also referred to Dr. Robert Young to be evaluated for antidepressants.

On August 26, 1993, the client was sent by her boss with a check to pay for an overdue mortgage payment on his condo. On the way back to work, the client was involved in an automobile accident. From that point on, her psychiatric symptoms worsened. She was experiencing anxiety, depression, nightmares, and fear of driving. By October of 1992, the client was fired from her job. She has not worked since then.

At the present time she spends most of her time at home. She claims that her mood fluctuates a great deal. She is often irritable and angry; she finds herself crying about minor issues and having problems with concentration. At the present time the client is under psychiatric care, for both psychotherapy and medication.

The psychological testing was requested to assess Ms. Silver's current cognitive and emotional characteristics as well as her personality structure.

During the clinical interview, the client came across as a bright and verbal woman who at times ran into difficulties in providing history, particularly in relation to the sequence of events. She made the effort to cooperate thoroughly with the various tasks, but showed concern about her performance. During the course of the evaluation, there were observable signs of anxiety, disappointment, and feelings of inadequacy. She admits to having suicidal ideations without the intent to carry. She claims that even during this evaluation she was "tuning out": "sometimes I don't hear what people tell me, my concentration and memory is not good anymore."

Psychological Report
Michelle Silver
3/14/94
Page 10 of 11

The integration of all the current testing data, the clinical evaluation, and the projective and objective testing reveal the following information about Ms. Silver. Her performance in the intelligence test indicates that she is currently functioning within the average range of intelligence. Furthermore, her overall pattern of IQ subtest scores presents a picture that is typical of a client with clinical depression and anxiety. Her results indicate a weakness in areas that relate to immediate memory, concentration, attention, visual, spatial ability, and speed, which are known to be lowered by anxiety or depression. Based on her results, in all probability, premorbidly, the client had functioned at a higher intellectual level.

Through the use of ambiguous stimuli, the projective tests elicit meaningful information about the individual's personality conflicts. Projective tests are less susceptible to faking and tend to reveal unconscious global aspects about the personality. Ms. Silver's projective data suggest that she has an intact ego in good contact with reality. They show that her quality of thinking is generally orderly and realistic. They further reveal that at the present time this client's tolerance of stress is rather limited. Furthermore, there were strong elements to suggest anxiety, depression, suspiciousness, worry, morbid themes, and concern about her future. On the other hand, the material also suggests that this individual is capable of entering into meaningful relationships and of seeing people interacting in a healthy way.

The client was given the MMPI at this office on two separate occasions, the first in October of 1993 and the second in March of 1994 during this current testing. Her profiles reveal similar findings. Her overall symptoms continued to present a picture of an individual who is significantly depressed, highly suspicious, and intensely worried about her health. Also, her results indicate that she is currently experiencing a high level of agitation, anxiety, and cognitive disorganization.

We are dealing here with a woman who, according to her history, has worked and supported herself from the time she was 15 years of age. Furthermore, she has continued to strive to improve herself, both with work and experience. She admits that in the past she has had episodes of mild depression and that she was able to get out of them rather quickly. However, by April of 1992, as a result of work-related stress, she began to exhibit significant symptoms of depression that included tearfulness, fatigue, irritability, weight gain, and poor concentration. She eventually sought psychiatric help.

The client's work history and the available medical records reveal nondisabling symptoms previous to the ones mentioned above. For the past year and a half, this client has been out of work and is suffering from both emotional and physical symptoms serious enough to interfere with every aspect of her life.

On a positive note, the client recognizes that therapy and medication have helped her, and she appears to be motivated to continue in the treatment. Furthermore, she shows strong interest in obtaining vocational rehabilitation to help her return to the labor market.

SAMPLE

Psychological Report
Michelle Silver
3/14/94
Page 11 of 11

DIAGNOSTIC IMPRESSIONS

AXIS I: 296.20—Major Depression, Single Episode. Symptoms include diminished concentration and memory, sleep disturbance, agitation, fatigue, sad mood, and decreased interest in normal activities.

AXIS II: No diagnosis.

AXIS III: Physical Disorder or Condition—Since the automobile accident in August of 1992, the client has been complaining of headaches and some numbness in her legs.

RECOMMENDATIONS

1. Both clinical and test evaluations indicate that Ms. Silver is experiencing significant emotional difficulties that include feelings of depression and anxiety. Because the client has already developed a good therapeutic relationship with her psychologist and psychiatrist, it is highly recommended that she continue to receive treatment, both for medication and psychotherapy, until things stabilize for her.

2. It is highly recommended that the client be given the opportunity for vocational rehabilitation. Returning her to the labor market would give her more purpose in life and improve her self-esteem, especially since this is an individual who has been working continually from the time she was 15 years of age.

It is hoped that this information will be helpful to you in the assessment of Ms. Michelle Silver's current psychological functioning. If you have any further questions, please feel free to contact me.

Very truly yours,

Cynthia Roberts, Ph.D.

CR/ab

Psychiatric Evaluation

The following psychiatric report is written by a forensic psychiatrist specializing in the treatment of posttraumatic stress disorders and mood disorders. Ms. Silver was referred to Dr. Young because of his specialization. The psychiatric report format used by Dr. Young contains the following sections:

1. Introductory Data

2. Current Complaints

3. History of Present Illness as Related by the Patient

4. Review of Records

5. Personal History

6. Medical History

7. Work History

8. Mental Status Exam

9. Psychological Testing

10. DSM-III-R Diagnosis

11. Summary and Discussion

12. Recommendations

Psychiatric Evaluation

SAMPLE

ROBERT YOUNG, M.D.
2201 Center Boulevard
Los Angeles, CA 90000
(213) 444-3333

April 21, 1994

David Stein
Attorney at Law
4625 Park Avenue
Los Angeles, CA 91234

> RE: Michelle Silver
> EMP: E & M Computers, Inc.
> WCAB: 92 ABC 1234
> D/I: C.T. 10/91—10/92
> D/E: 10/8/93; 4/21/94

PSYCHIATRIC EVALUATION

Dear Mr. Stein:

The following is a report of an extended evaluation of the above-named patient that took place on two occasions. This evaluation was conducted for medical-legal purposes. It includes a detailed history, mental status exam, results of routine psychological testing, findings, discussion, recommendations, and assessment of disability. Medical records that were available are herein reviewed. The patient was evaluated by me.

INTRODUCTORY DATA

Ms. Michelle Silver is a 35-year-old woman who was employed by E & M Computers, Inc., as a bookkeeper from January 1991 to October 1992. The patient experienced a great deal of emotional stress during the course of her employment and was involved in an automobile accident while working for this employer. She has developed severe psychiatric symptomatology, for which she has received treatment. The purpose of this current evaluation is to ascertain the connection between the patient's current psychiatric problems and the industrial stressors.

CURRENT COMPLAINTS

Emotional

1. Depressive symptoms: She states that she is depressed most of the time and has become, at times, totally immobilized and unable to make decisions for herself. She is frequently tearful and has minimal interest in socialization and other activities. She describes low self-esteem, easy fatigability, decreased concentration, decreased memory and low libido.

2. Anxiety symptoms: She frequently feels anxious. She has sleep disturbance, waking up in

Psychiatric Evaluation
Michelle Silver
4/21/94
Page 2 of 11

the middle of the night several times and early in the morning. She also feels more angry and irritable than is usual for her. She describes having, at times, "anxiety attacks."

Physical

1. Headaches: "I get them about three times a week . . . before it was every day. I take Fiorinal when I need to."

2. Gastrointestinal problems: "I get stomach aches, cramps, gas . . . . This is a problem daily."

3. Backaches: "I get low back pain mainly in the mornings . . . maybe it's related to the stomach problems."

4. Leg pain: She describes numbness in her legs, as well as pain in her feet, which required minor surgery.

HISTORY OF PRESENT ILLNESS AS RELATED BY THE PATIENT

The patient began working for E & M Computers, Inc. as a bookkeeper in January 1991. She reports being in good physical and mental health at the time she was hired. She states that her employer, Mr. Fred Miller, is the company's owner.

She states that it was immediately obvious that "they're very poorly organized . . . no system there . . . roaches in the office . . . papers everywhere . . . dark, depressing place . . . but there were nice people working there."

But, she says, she "saw it as a challenge . . . I rearranged and organized things . . . I put in a lot of overtime without pay . . . I started finding mistakes and things that had been stolen . . . felt he appreciated my input."

She described Mr. Miller as having some interpersonal problems with the employees in that "he often yelled and cursed." She recalls first having problems with him as early as March of 1991. "He had a habit of not paying things . . . employee's checks would bounce . . . I'd try to rectify the situation . . . he would yell at me . . . sometimes I went home crying."

"I was the one who got the call from people who were angry . . . people whose gas and lights had been turned off . . . mortgage not paid . . . I'd feel my hands were tied as far as paying the bills . . . there was nothing I could do . . . on a daily basis he would scream and throw things . . . not at us but at the wall or in the air . . . and swear."

"There would be good and bad days . . . sometimes I'd have to do a lot of driving to go pay bills at the last minute . . . it could have all been avoided . . . It got worse after my friend quit in September . . . she had helped to keep some of the pressure off of me . . . we [the office] were also evicted and had to move . . . there was a lot of reorganization and work . . . a lot of people were fired because of lack of funds . . . the work load increased."

The patient states that she considered looking for another job, but felt she had financial responsibilities and no time to do job interviewing. By approximately April or May of 1992,

Psychiatric Evaluation
Michelle Silver
4/21/94
Page 3 of 11

she felt that the pressure had finally become overwhelming. "I wasn't sleeping well . . . I was waking up every two hours . . . I started hating the place . . . I was coming in late . . . I guess I was looking to get fired without realizing it . . . I gained about 20 pounds . . . I was irritable and not socializing . . . friends noticed a change in me . . . I'd cry when he yelled . . . I was tired and nervous . . . I wasn't concentrating well."

The patient states that her symptoms increased further when the company moved a second time in June 1992. "Everybody was in one room . . . there was no privacy and it was very hard to work . . . my boss was going through a divorce and he'd yell at me and other people when he was upset. It was very bad . . . he had a lawsuit against him for being a slumlord . . . it made it even worse at work and there was more pressure there."

The patient gives another example, occurring in August 1992, of the ongoing frustrating interaction she had with her employer. "For a week prior to my automobile accident I warned him that his mortgage was due . . . he was always yelling at me . . . and he had me go at the last minute to make the mortgage payment . . . that's when I had my car accident." The accident occurred on August 26, 1992, in the bank's parking lot. "I was hit head-on . . . there were obstacles that made it hard to see around the corner . . . I had a lump on the left side of my head . . . I lost a week of work."

She states that after her automobile accident her depression reached the point where "I just didn't care anymore. When I returned to work, I was daydreaming and working short hours . . . I felt very angry about the accident . . . it was so hard to be at work . . . I felt like there was no way out." At that point her anxiety symptoms became out of control, and she began to have nightmares as well as serious physical symptoms with severe headaches, dizziness, muscle spasms, stiffness in her neck, extreme physical tension, and tearfulness.

The patient was terminated from her job in October 1992 "because I wasn't efficient anymore." She has not worked since that time.

The patient sought treatment with Dr. George R. Jones for psychotherapy on a once-a-week basis. She states she initiated treatment with him in April 1992 as her depressive and anxious symptomatology became worse.

Dr. George Jones, her therapist, then referred the patient to me to ascertain the need for medications, i.e., antidepressants and anxiolytics. I have been managing the patient's medications including Norpramin, Tofranil, Desyrel, and Nardil (antidepressants). She has also been tried on Xanax, Lithium, and Navane. There have been a lot of ups and downs during the course of her treatment, and she has had difficulty tolerating many of the medications.

Most recently, the patient has been maintained on a dose of Norpramin, 250 milligrams a day.

Because of the neurologic symptoms that developed after the automobile accident, and the head trauma, I felt it was necessary to send this patient for a neurological consultation. She saw Irene Phillips, M.D. She has treated her for the postconcussive and muscle-contraction headaches as well as other neurologic sequelae of the automobile accident.

Psychiatric Evaluation
Michelle Silver
4/21/94
Page 4 of 11

The patient has attended her psychotherapy as well as her psychiatric appointments regularly and has been extremely cooperative in taking her medication. Because of the severity of the depressive and anxious symptomatology, she has not been able to reenter the labor market despite a very strong desire to do so.

The patient has made some attempts to enter vocational rehabilitation, but because of intermittent worsening of her depressive symptoms, this has been very hard for her to pursue.

The patient openly acknowledges that although she feels she is making some progress, she is still having significant emotional problems. She does not feel ready to reenter the labor market, noting, "I still don't feel ready... I'm afraid to work ... I'm not even sure what I want to do ... I feel lost."

REVIEW OF RECORDS

Report on diagnosis and impression to Dr. Irene Phillips dated September 30, 1992:

1. Postconcussive headache, acute. This patient has had a marked increase in headaches after her motor vehicle accident approximately one month ago. These seem to be improving slowly, and the patient treats them intermittently with Fiorinal with codeine. I will give the patient a trial of Midrin as a nonnarcotic analgesic, which may be helpful during these headaches.

2. Tension/muscle-contraction headaches, chronic. This appears to be a chronic problem. It is probably exacerbated by the patient's current depressed mood. I have discussed with the patient the likely improvement in these headaches when her mood improves, but in the interim she will attempt to treat these headaches with relaxation techniques and Midrin, if needed.

3. Blepharospasm.

4. Meralgia paresthetica.

5. Tinnitus.

Report of Dr. Phillips dated October 21, 1992:

1. Postconcussive headaches: These seem to be resolving without treatment. No further evaluation is planned.

2. Tension/muscle-contraction headache: These continue to plague the patient and are probably exacerbated by the patient's current depressed mood, although this seems better. She will continue to use her relaxation techniques and Midrin.

3. Blepharospasm: This problem is resolved for her.

4. Meralgia paresthetica: This is bilateral, but today seems more prominent on the left. No further evaluation is planned.

Psychiatric Evaluation
Michelle Silver
4/21/94
Page 5 of 11

5. Tinnitus: The patient's brainstem auditory evoked response was normal. No further evaluation is planned.

PERSONAL HISTORY

The patient was born and raised in Oregon. She states that she moved with her family to California at the age of 15.

She states that she has two sisters and five brothers. One of her brothers died in an automobile accident in 1988. She is the second youngest of her siblings.

Her father is 75 years old and described as being in good health. He worked in the Army for 17 years and then as a driver. He is described as "a very military-like person . . . very self-dependent. I think he's getting a little senile now . . . it's hard to be patient with him since I have such a low tolerance now."

Her mother is 65 years old. She states that her mother has primarily been a homemaker although she has also done some laundry and sewing work. She is a foster parent to three children. "She always complains about her health but she's a strong person."

She states that she has a rather poor memory of her childhood. "My father was working much of the time and summer was spent at summer camp . . . but I feel there wasn't enough communication and love in my family."

She graduated high school. She states that she completed some college classes but did not receive a degree. She did get a certificate from business college in accounting.

The patient has had some long-term relationships. She states that she has dated and recently ended a relationship with a man that she had been seeing for approximately nine months.

MEDICAL HISTORY

The patient had a tonsillectomy at the age of 7. She was hospitalized for one week due to infection.

She had gall bladder surgery at the age of 22.

At the age of 25 she had surgery on her feet.

She states that she has a history of thrombophlebitis dating back to 1973.

She has had two bladder infections occurring in July 1991 and January 1992. One bladder infection led to brief hospitalization.

She had two abortions, at the ages of 19 and 30.

She denies any allergies. She drinks approximately one cup of coffee daily. She rarely drinks alcohol.

She states that she stopped smoking cigarettes one year ago. Prior to that time she smoked approximately one pack every week or two.

Psychiatric Evaluation
Michelle Silver
4/21/94
Page 6 of 11

Her current medication includes Norpramin, 250 milligrams, and Fiorinal with codeine, for headaches.

The patient first received psychotherapy with Dr. George R. Jones in 1992, when she was having depressive symptomatology as a consequence of problems with her supervisor, Mr. Miller. She states that she felt this depression continued but was much less severe than her current depression. She denies any other history of mental illness or psychotherapy.

WORK HISTORY

From 1974 to 1976 the patient worked at St. Mary's Hospital in Torrance, while receiving nursing training. From 1976 to 1985, she worked for St. Mary's Hospital in the nursing department.

She attended accounting school during 1984. She then obtained a job with a management company as an accountant, which she held from 1985 to 1988.

She then left her job to attend school to be a travel agent. After completing part of the training, she discontinued when her brother died.

She worked as a bookkeeper for an electronics company from 1990 to 1991. When this company went out of business, she obtained her most recent job with E & M Computers, Inc. in January 1991.

MENTAL STATUS EXAM

General Description: The patient is a casually dressed woman looking her stated age. She is cooperative with the examiner. She is a good historian.

Speech: She spoke in a normal tone with good vocabulary.

State of Consciousness: The patient was alert and able to carry out simple and complex orders.

Mood: She admits to feeling sad, anxious, and worried about the future.

Affect: The patient's affect is quite sad and congruent with the stated mood.

Stream of Thought: There is no formal thought disorder.

Content of Thought: There is much focus on her feelings of sadness, inadequacy, confusion, and lack of direction.

Perception: There are no visual or auditory hallucinations.

Orientation: The patient is well-oriented to self, place, and time.

Memory: The patient has some difficulty with tasks of memory but is able to recall dates fairly well.

Information and Intelligence: Average

Concentration: She has limited concentration and had difficulty on tasks of concentration.

Abstract Thinking: Ability to think abstractly is relatively intact.

Psychiatric Evaluation
Michelle Silver
4/21/94
Page 7 of 11

Judgment: Gross and test judgment are intact.

Insight: The patient has some insight into her own emotional dynamics but continues to function at a rather low level.

PSYCHOLOGICAL TESTING

Bender Gestalt Perceptual Motor Functioning Test: Reproduction of configurations was adequate and revealed no gross organic brain dysfunction.

Beck Depression Inventory: This is a self-rating scale for depression. The patient's score reflects significant depression. Positive findings include: feeling so sad or unhappy that it is quite painful; feeling that she won't ever get over her troubles; feeling she has accomplished very little that is worthwhile; not enjoying things the way she used to; feeling as though she is bad or worthless; having the feeling that something bad might happen; being disappointed in herself; being critical of herself for her weaknesses; having thoughts of harming herself, although she would not carry them out; feeling annoyed or irritated more easily than she used to; having much less interest in other people than she used to; having great difficulty in making decisions; not working as well as she used to; fatiguing more easily than she used to; having less interest in sex than she used to; and being concerned about various aches and pains.

Hamilton Psychiatric Rating Scale for Depression: This is scored by the examiner, based on observations and questioning. The Hamilton reflects significant depressive symptomatology, with depressed mood reflected verbally and nonverbally, including feelings of guilt, profound sleep disturbance, loss of interest in usual activities, retardation intermixed with agitation, psychic and somatic anxiety, feelings of heaviness, diminished sexual interest, markedly increased suspiciousness, and obsessional thinking.

Sentence Completion Test: The majority of the patient's responses reflect her feelings of sadness, anger, mistrust of people, and negativism about the future. Positive findings include: It hurts when "someone uses me." In ten years, "what have I accomplished?" No one knows "what I feel inside." When I am alone, "I think." I find it hard to decide "what to do." Nothing is harder to stop than "your feelings." I used to daydream "about a happy time." When I am criticized, "I hurt." When a job seems impossible, "I get sick and depressed." Sometimes your best friend will "hurt you." I cannot stand "unfairness." I find it hard to fall asleep "when I have a problem." My sexual drive "is slow." When I am in a large crowd, "I feel lost." When I am ill, "I feel sad." There ought to be a law "against users." The thing that embarrasses me most is "being insulted in public."

Review of MMPI Scored and Interpreted by Cynthia Roberts, Ph.D.: The patient obtained a valid profile indicating that "at the present time she is highly suspicious; she may be experiencing some difficulty with people in authority, and she is highly agitated, significantly depressed, intensely worried about her health, highly anxious, and is undergoing some

Psychiatric Evaluation
Michelle Silver
4/21/94
Page 8 of 11

cognitive disorganization. Furthermore, because of her current distress, her perception of reality is rather tenuous." The profile reflects a great deal of anger and of difficulty in expressing it. Dr. Roberts suggested a therapy that is supportive in nature.

DSM-III-R DIAGNOSIS

Axis I: 296.20 Major depression. Single episode with sad mood, loss of interest in usual activities, weight gain, insomnia, psychomotor agitation, fatigue, feelings of worthlessness, diminished concentration, and tearfulness.

309.89 Posttraumatic stress disorder. Symptoms include history of recurrent recollections of the event, nightmares, fear of being injured, diminished interest in activities, sleep disturbance, irritability, difficulty concentrating, hypervigilance, and exaggerated startle response.

Axis II: Personality diagnosis. No diagnosis, but there are some obsessive-compulsive and masochistic features.

Axis III: Physical disorder or condition. History of head trauma in automobile accident (August 26, 1992), history of headaches subsequent to the accident.

SUMMARY AND DISCUSSION

Ms. Michelle Silver is a 35-year-old woman who worked for E & M Computers, Inc. as a bookkeeper from January 1991 to October 1992.

The patient states that she immediately noticed problems at her workplace, including poor organization, disorder, and a work setting that was dark, poorly ventilated, and had many cockroaches.

While the patient states her coworkers were "very nice people," she found that her employer, Mr. George Miller, yelled and cursed at employees a great deal. By March 1991, she states that she was already feeling he was misdirecting anger at her. Typically, Mr. Miller would not pay his bills nor allow enough money in his account to cover payroll or other important costs. When the patient would try to rectify this situation, Mr. Miller would become angry. The patient repeatedly took verbal abuse from various account holders who were angry with her employer.

"I was the one who had to field the calls . . . I was yelled at . . . there was nothing I could do . . . People were having their gas and lights turned off . . . the mortgage wasn't being paid . . . he would have me drive at the last minute to pay bills . . . I worked a lot of overtime."

The patient feels her work stress increased after a coworker quit in September 1991. "She had helped me . . . taken some pressure off me." Near that same time, she states that the office had to be moved because her employer was evicted for not paying his bills. Many of her coworkers were fired, and she feels that a great deal of responsibility for moving and reorganizing things fell upon her.

Psychiatric Evaluation
Michelle Silver
4/21/94
Page 9 of 11

The patient described trying to look at the job "as a challenge," but becoming increasingly distressed with the situation. While she considered looking elsewhere for work, she felt that financial pressures and time limits for job hunting did not allow her to do this.

By April 1992, she was beginning to exhibit symptoms of depression including sleep disturbance, sad mood, tearfulness, social withdrawal, fatigue, irritability, weight gain, anxiety, decreased sexual drive, and decreased concentration. At that point she sought psychotherapy from Dr. George Jones. She was still maintaining herself at her job, but her ability to function was becoming very tenuous.

At that point Dr. Jones referred the patient to me for psychopharmacologic intervention, i.e., he felt that she was suffering from a major depression and that she needed antidepressants. Various medications were tried. Unfortunately, the patient had some difficulty in tolerating some of the antidepressant medications earlier on.

The symptoms of depression continued to increase as additional work pressures were put on her. She states that her employer was going through a divorce, and she felt that he often took his anger out on her and the other employees. There was another move of her office in June 1992 in which "everyone was in one room." She described that the lack of privacy exacerbated the already existing problems.

The patient recalls that in August 1992 she had warned her employer over a one-week period regarding having to pay his mortgage. She states that as he typically did, he waited until the last minute, requiring her to do unnecessary driving. While going to her employer's bank, she was in an automobile accident. She suffered an injury to her head and was treated. She was off work for one week.

Unfortunately, after the automobile accident her symptoms became much worse and she developed a full-blown posttraumatic stress disorder with nightmares, some fear of driving, extreme anxiety, irritability, a further diminished concentration, and difficulty in being around other people.

Because of the postconcussive symptoms, including severe headaches and severe muscle tension, I felt that she needed to see a neurologist and thus referred her to Irene Phillips, M.D., who diagnosed her as having "postconcussive headaches . . . tension muscle-contraction headaches . . . blepharospasm . . . meralgia paresthetica and tinnitus." The patient began to receive medications for these headaches.

I feel that the patient had already developed symptoms that met the DSM-III-R criteria for a major depression prior to her automobile accident. The automobile accident served to further exacerbate an already serious depression, leading to very poor work performance and apathy, and resulting in her job termination on October 10, 1992.

I believe the automobile accident precipitated additional symptoms that meet the DSM-III-R criteria for posttraumatic stress disorder. Specifically, the patient had some recurrent recollections of the accident, nightmares, fear of being hurt, severe sleep disturbance,

Psychiatric Evaluation
Michelle Silver
4/21/94
Page 10 of 11

irritability, hypervigilance, and exaggerated startle response.

It is possible that without the automobile accident the patient may have been able to maintain herself in some employment with the help of medications and psychotherapy; however, after this automobile accident, she totally decompensated in her progress in psychiatric and psychotherapeutic treatment and since August 1992 has been extremely slow.

The patient has been receiving psychotherapy for her depression with Dr. George Jones, Ph.D. since April 1992. I have been managing her medication since May 1992. The course of her treatment has had a lot of ups and downs. We have tried several medications, and she appears to gain the most benefit from her current medication, Norpramin, 250 milligrams a day. Unfortunately, this medication has not brought a remission of her severe depression; however, without the medication her symptoms are even worse.

While her posttraumatic stress disorder symptoms have improved, her depression is still quite severe and seriously interfering with her functioning in all spheres. As an example, she canceled her first scheduled appointment for this evaluation and would have not shown up on October 8 if I had not called her and encouraged her to come in. It seemed very difficult for her to go over what had happened at her job and to go over the events of the automobile accident. She has extreme difficulty getting up in the morning and motivating herself to do things.

The only positive thing that has occurred recently is that she has shown a strong interest in vocational rehabilitation, despite the ongoing symptomatology. Given this patient's strong work ethic and motivation to return to the labor market, I feel we should help her as much as we can in this endeavor. I feel that if she were helped to return to the labor market, some of her self-esteem would return. However, unfortunately, we are looking at a very hard road ahead for this young woman, given the up-and-down nature of her current depressive illness. I feel that the work-related stress and the automobile accident led to a fragmentation of her ego defenses, and I can honestly say that it has taken a great deal of effort to try to put this patient back together.

In summary, I feel this patient developed a major depression as a result of the emotional stress at her workplace. Her depression did not become disabling until after the added stressor of an automobile accident. The automobile accident also added an overlay of posttraumatic stress disorder. There are no significant nonindustrial psychosocial stressors to which these psychiatric problems can be attributed. Although this patient relates some past history of mild depression, there is no previous history of any severe depressions and no psychiatrically related disability previously.

RECOMMENDATIONS

I strongly feel that this patient should continue to receive psychiatric treatment, including psychotherapy and antidepressant and anxiolytic medications. It has already been noted that

Psychiatric Evaluation
Michelle Silver
4/21/94
Page 11 of 11

when the patient was taken off her medication, her symptoms were significantly exacerbated.
I that feel this patient will also need vocational counseling and rehabilitation to reenter the
labor market successfully.

Sincerely,

Robert Young, M.D.

RY/mg

Conclusion

In conclusion, I want to remind you, as always, that *you're the doctor.* Although these forms and formats have been field-tested for years, you are the best judge of your paperwork needs and you may want to modify the forms to suit your unique practice. What these forms offer you is a *structure* for the documentation process.

As you use these forms, you may find that certain forms or formats are useful on a daily basis, while others may be used rarely in the general course of your clinical practice. Whether you use a form once or a thousand times, having it there to draw on saves you time, thought, and energy. Ultimately, our hope is that these forms will save you countless organizational hours, so that you can spend more time focused on clinical work—the meaningful work we therapists do.

Laws and ethics change, and the requirements for the continuing treatment of patients under health insurance plans will always be in a dynamic state of flux. As there are significant changes in administrative systems, we will revise this book and the forms and reports. We welcome your comments and suggestions so that we may improve the forms wherever possible to suit your real needs.

We look forward to your contributions and hope that ours have made your professional life that much easier.

Index

TO CUSTOMIZE YOUR FORMS SEND FOR THIS PERSONALIZED OVERLAY TODAY!

SIMPLY TAKE THE CLEAR PLASTIC OVERLAY WITH YOUR CUSTOMIZED LETTERHEAD ON IT,

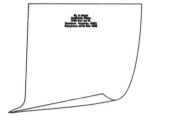

+

PHOTOCOPY IT OVER THE PREPRINTED FORMS FROM THE BOOK,

=

AND YOU HAVE A PERSONALIZED FORM FOR YOUR OFFICE!

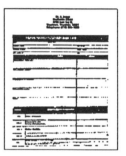

CHOOSE FROM SIX DISTINCTIVE TYPEFACES

Arial
Dr. A. Jones
Northside Clinic
3700 East 3rd Street
Yourtown, Yourstate 10000
Telephone (212) 555-5000

Bahamas
Dr. A. Jones
Northside Clinic
3700 East 3rd Street
Yourtown, Yourstate 10000
Telephone (212) 555-5000

Bodoni
Dr. A. Jones
Northside Clinic
3700 East 3rd Street
Yourtown, Yourstate 10000
Telephone (212) 555-5000

Bookman
Dr. A. Jones
Northside Clinic
3700 East 3rd Street
Yourtown, Yourstate 10000
Telephone (212) 555-5000

Gill Sans
Dr. A. Jones
Northside Clinic
3700 East 3rd Street
Yourtown, Yourstate 10000
Telephone (212) 555-5000

Stone Serif
Dr. A. Jones
Northside Clinic
3700 East 3rd Street
Yourtown, Yourstate 10000
Telephone (212) 555-5000

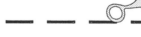

Send a check for twenty-five dollars ($25)* to:
GMS
P.O. Box 1907
Redondo Beach, CA 90278
Or pay by VISA ( ) or Mastercard ( )
Card number _____
Expiration date _____
Name as it appears on card _____
Signature of cardholder _____
Ship To:
Name _____
Address _____
City/ State / Zip _____
Telephone _____
*CA residents add $2.13 sales tax

Information for Personalized Overlay
Physician Name _____
Clinic Name _____
Address(es) _____
_____
Telephone number(s) _____
Type of License _____
License number _____

Select Typeface:
☐ Arial   ☐ Bookman
☐ Bahamas   ☐ Gill Sans
☐ Bodoni   ☐ Stone Serif

Crisis and Bibliotherapy Resources

CRISIS RESOURCES

TRAUMA IN THE LIVES OF CHILDREN: Crisis and Stress Management Techniques for Counselors and Other Professionals
by Kendall Johnson, Ph.D.

Children may suffer trauma at any age: from a natural disaster, violence in the home, or seeing a shooting at school. If not properly handled, the trauma will have lasting effects on the child's development. In this practical book for professionals who work with children in crisis, Dr. Johnson provides effective guidelines to prepare for and handle a crisis, and identify traumatized children who need help.
256 pages ... Paperback ... $15.95

SCHOOL CRISIS MANAGEMENT: A Team Training Guide
by Kendall Johnson, Ph.D.

Written for school professionals—administrators, psychologists, counselors, and crisis response team members—this detailed guide goes beyond introductory trauma theory to give practical applications, specific procedures, and proven strategies for managing crisis situations in schools. Includes 78 full-page charts that may be copied to make overhead transparencies.
192 pages ... 78 illus ... Paperback $19.95 ... Spiral $24.95

BIBLIOTHERAPY RESOURCES

WHEN SOMEONE YOU LOVE IS IN THERAPY
by Michael Gold, Ph.D., with Marie Scampini

Explains the ins and outs of therapy to those whose loved ones are going through it, and answers such questions as "Why did they go into therapy?" "What goes on there?" "How do I know if something goes wrong?" and "What about me?" This book demystifies psychotherapy and shows readers how to cope with their *own* feelings—their questions, fears, anxieties, and insecurities—so they can feel confident themselves and be supportive of their loved one.
208 pages ... Paperback ... $10.95

TURNING YOURSELF AROUND: Self-Help for Troubled Teens
by Kendall Johnson, Ph.D.

This is a support book for young adults, ages 15–20, who are going through 12-step programs. It follows the stories of three young people—one a bulimic, another an alcoholic, and the third a relationship addict. We see their individual problems, personal needs, and different stages of recovery. The book provides overviews of the issues, followed by provocative questions and exercises that will help all teens deal with life issues. A pullout guide for parents, teachers, or counselors is included.
224 pages ... Paperback ... $9.95

SEXUAL HEALING: A Self-Help Program to Enhance Your Sensuality and Overcome Common Sexual Problems
by Barbara Keesling, Ph.D.

Dr. Keesling gives expert advice on how to overcome common sexual problems. Using her experience as both a surrogate partner and a sex therapist, Dr. Keesling offers a program of exercises to effectively eliminate problems such as: performance anxiety, premature ejaculation, inhibited ejaculation, erection problems, low desire issues, and inability to achieve orgasm.

Sensate focus is the basis of the exercises in *Sexual Healing*—touching for your own pleasure and focusing on the exact point of touch. These techniques have been proven to work on thousands of clients.

The book includes: **Part I:** introductory material on surrogate partners, sexuality, health; **Part II:** how to recognize sexual problems; **Part III:** how to approach the exercises and focus; **Part IV:** basic exercises and common barriers; **Interlude:** optional playful sexual activities; **Part V:** advanced exercises for specific sexual problems; **Part VI:** adding mutuality to sexual contact.
288 pages ... Paperback ... $12.95

GROWTH AND RECOVERY WORKBOOKS
by Wendy Deaton, MFCC and Kendall Johnson, Ph.D.

The *Growth and Recovery Workbooks* are a series of clinical tools written by a family counselor and an expert in psychotraumatology to help professionals in their work with children. In one place they provide a medium for care that is creative and can be tailored to the child's needs.

The layout of the books is open and encouraging. Each page has an exercise or task keyed to the phases and goals of therapy, and invites the child to express himself or herself freely. Tasks are balanced between writing and drawing, left and right brain, thought and feeling.

The *Growth and Recovery Workbooks* are not self-help tools. They come with a therapist's guide and are intended to be used by professionals only, in a confidential setting. Using these Workbooks can help to:

- provide a focus, develop communication and trust
- reduce anxiety and correct misconceptions
- invite children to explore their whole range of thoughts and feelings
- identify the strengths, skills, and support network they already have

The workbooks are also available as Practitioner Packs, each containing one workbook, the therapist's guide, and reproductions of each exercise on double-sided cards. These allow the therapist to make multiple copies or select individual task sequences for each child.

WORKBOOKS IN THE SERIES

Living with My Family (ages 9–12) is a workbook for children who have been traumatized by domestic violence or family quarrels. (Title code LWF)

No More Hurt (ages 9–12) is a workbook for children who have been physically, sexually, or psychologically abused. (Title code NMH)

A Separation in My Family (ages 9–12) is a workbook for children whose parents are separating or have been separated or divorced. (Title code SMF)

Someone I Love Died (ages 9–12) is a workbook about loss and grieving for children who have lost a loved one. (Title code SLD)

Drinking and Drugs in My Family (ages 9–12) is for working with children who have family members who are chemically dependent or engage in regular substance abuse. (Title code DDF)

My Own Thoughts (for Young Girls) (ages 7–10) is an exploratory workbook for girls who have problems with self-esteem, depression, conflict, maladjustment, and suspected trauma. (Title code MOT/G)

My Own Thoughts (for Young Boys) (ages 7–10) is an exploratory workbook for boys who have problems with self-esteem, depression, conflict, maladjustment, and suspected trauma. (Title code MOT/B)

My Own Thoughts On Stopping the Hurt (ages 7–10) is an exploratory workbook for working with young children where there is suspected physical or sexual abuse. (Title code MOT/H)

A selection of Behavioral Science Book Service

Current prices of workbooks and practitioner packs:

	Individual titles	Mixed titles
Single Workbooks	$5.95	
10-pack	$40.00 ($4.00/each)	$45.00 ($4.50/each)
50-pack	$180.00 ($3.60/each)	$200.00 ($4.00/each)
Practitioner Packs	$15.95 each	

——— SEND ME ——— ORDER FORM ——— SHIP TO ———

Title Code	Circle one	Price	Qty	Amount
	Bk / Pk			
	Bk / Pk			
	Bk / Pk			
	Bk / Pk			
	Bk / Pk			
	Bk / Pk			
	Bk / Pk			
	Bk / Pk			
In California add 7¼% sales tax				
Shipping and handling ($2.50 1st book, $.75 each add'l)				
TOTAL ENCLOSED				

FPP2A 3/94

Name _____

Organization _____

Street _____

City/State _____ Zip _____

Phone number (for credit card orders) _____

☐ Check ☐ Visa ☐ MC

Card # _____ Exp date _____

Signature _____

Hunter House Inc. Publishers • P.O. Box 2914 • Alameda CA 94501
For quantity discounts and shipping rates call 510/865-5282 or FAX 510/865-4295